AF207287

TALES FROM THE TRAILS

Previous books by Michael Clinton include:

American Portraits

Wanderlust

Global Faces

Global Remains

Global Snaps

The Globetrotter Diaries

Closer

Santa Fe

The Hamptons

TALES FROM THE TRAILS

Runners' Stories that Inspire and Transform

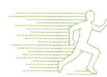

MICHAEL CLINTON

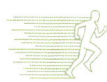

Foreword by Michael Capiraso   Preface by Jordan Metzl, MD

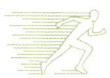

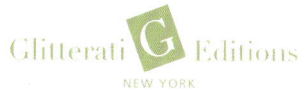

Glitterati G Editions
NEW YORK

First published in 2019 by

Glitterati Editions
311 West 43 Street
12th Floor
New York, NY 10036

www.glitteratieditions.com
media@glitteratieditions.com

Copyright © 2019 by Michael Clinton

All rights reserved. No part of this publication may be reproduced in any
form or by any electronic or mechanical means, including information
storage and retrieval systems, without permission in writing from the
publisher, except by a reviewer who may quote brief passages in a review.

First edition, 2019

Library of Congress Cataloging-in-Publication data
is available from the publisher.

Hardcover edition
ISBN: 978-1-943876-61-7

Printed and bound in China

10 9 8 7 6 5 4 3 2 1

Cover Photography Credits:
Center © Susie Noddle
Lower left © Laurel Abusamra
Upper right and page 147 © Ben Ko

This book is dedicated to my sister, Peg,
for her courage and stamina in running and in life.

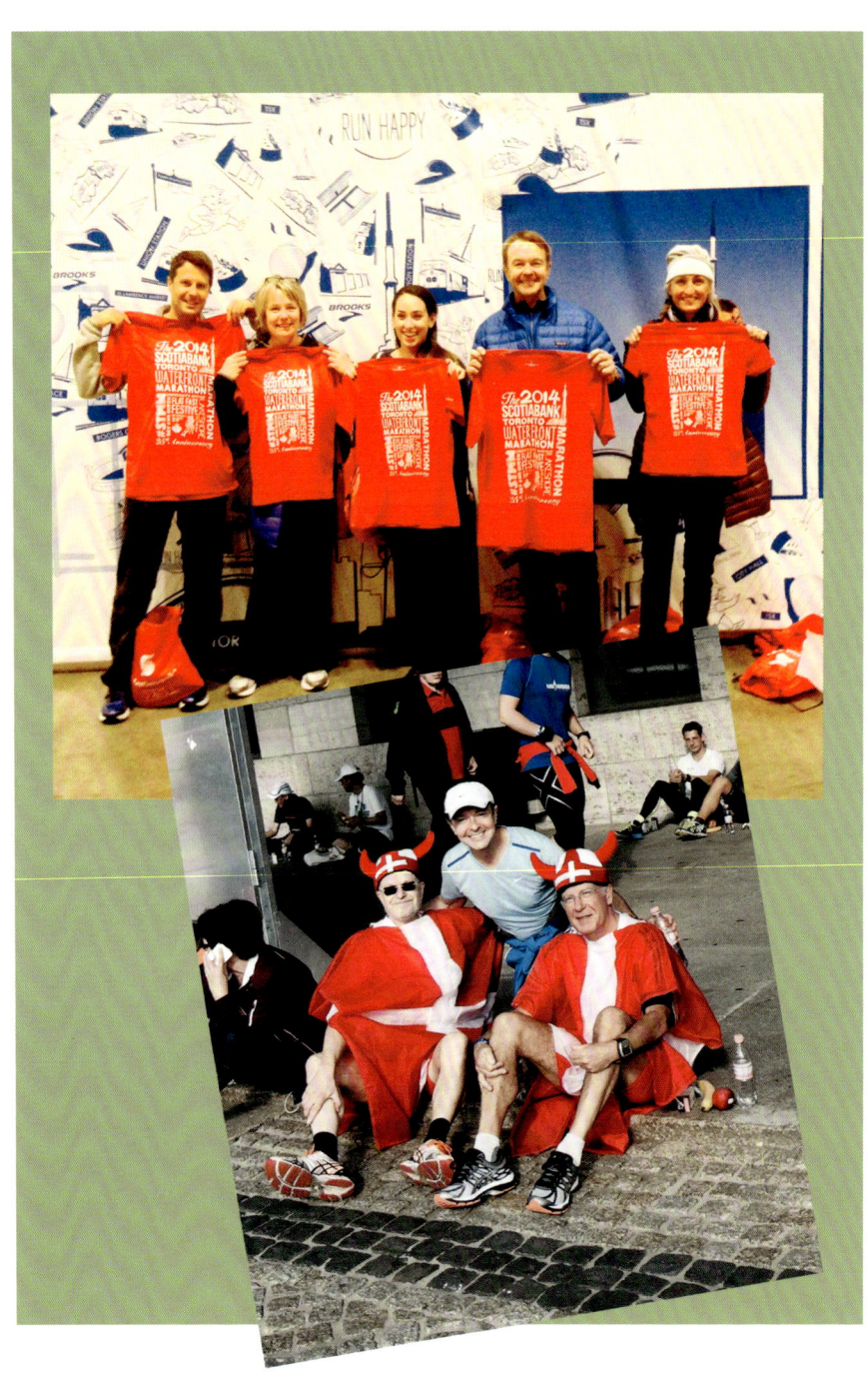

Contents

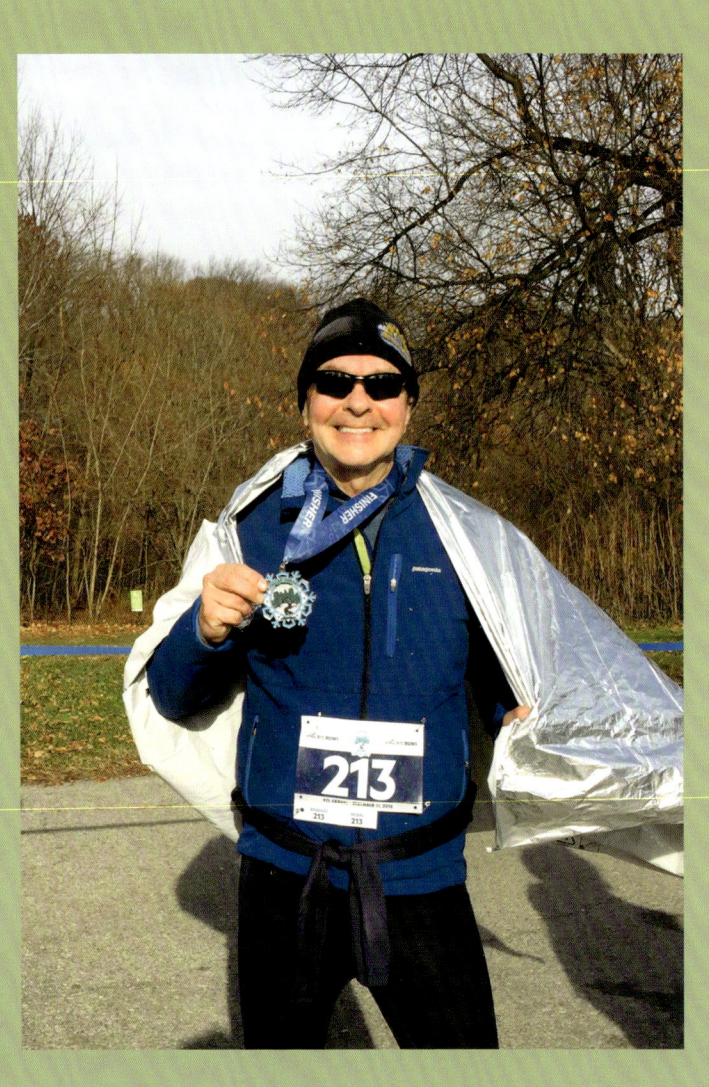

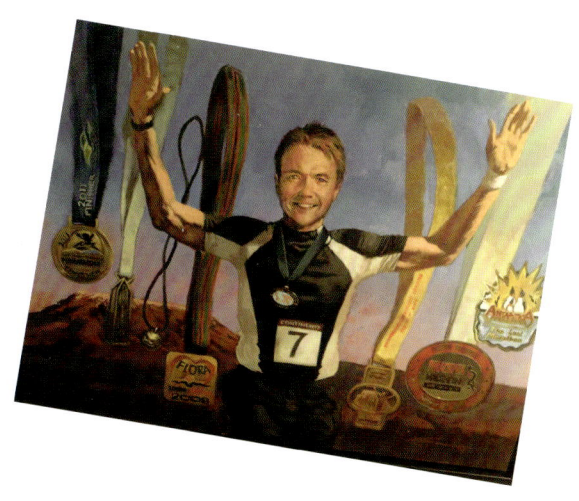

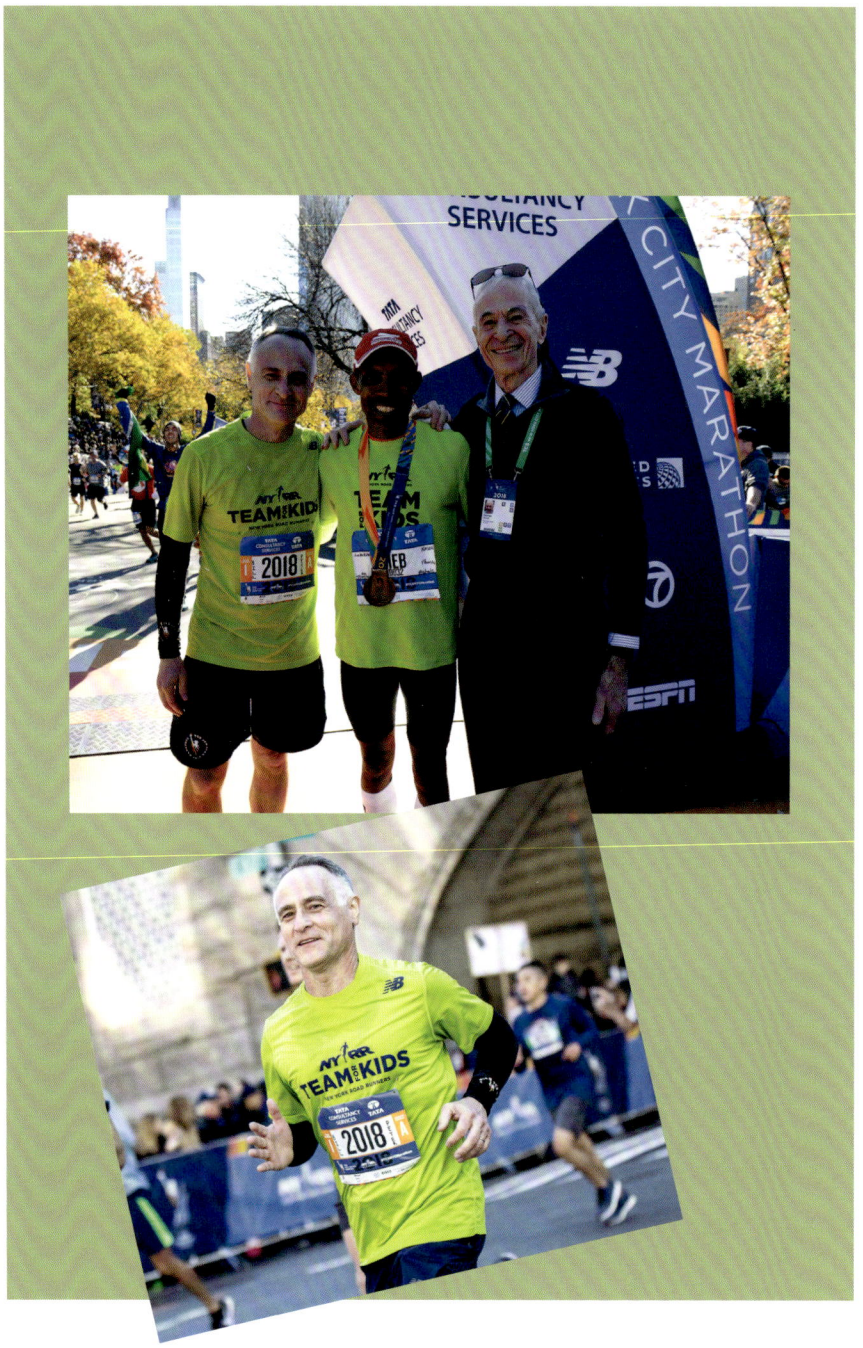

Foreword

Running

Michael Capiraso

We all find our own paths to becoming runners, our own inspirations to continue pushing forward and challenging ourselves. For some, running can be a connector, for some an escape, for some it's a way to prove something to the world, and for others it's a way to prove something to themselves.

The story of how I found running isn't unique, but it's certainly meaningful; an event in my life triggered me to go from a "sometimes runner" to "I need to RUN . . . I want to RUN!"

Twenty-eight years ago, I was dumped by my longtime girlfriend, and I was devastated. I said, "I'll show her; I'll run the New York City Marathon and she'll think I'm an amazing person with such discipline and courage, to set a goal as insurmountable as 26.2 miles and prove myself by achieving it and she'll take me back." I was inspired, though maybe a bit misguided when signing up for the 1991 New York City Marathon.

Well, I signed up, lined up, and ran up to the finish line of the 1991 NYC Marathon, and despite it all, I didn't win her back—actually, I never saw her again. But I crossed the finish line in Central Park, gaining a new experience and a new perspective. It brought me to a sport and lifestyle that has forever changed me: personally and professionally, mentally and physically. The impact of that fortuitous decision has been immeasurable and lifelong. It also, eventually, gave me the rare chance and perspective to utter the phrase, "Best breakup ever!"

This journey at that point in my life inspired me to make a change and fall in love with running. Most of us can anchor our running back to some major catalyst, and this was mine. What is unique to my story is that I thought the catalyst was my ex-girlfriend, and it took many years to realize that the catalyst was my lack of direction at that time in my life. While I was convinced this feat would cause a change of heart and lead to me winning her back, what it did instead, thankfully, was redirect me. It gave me running as part of a foundation for many aspects of my life that were now on course for growth, happiness, and many adventurous miles.

Throughout the subsequent twenty-eight years, running has led me down nearly every path in New York City and throughout the five boroughs: daily runs along the bridle path in Central Park, around the globe in Flushing Meadows Corona Park, the Coney Island Boardwalk, and of course, I've run at every destination that I've traveled to around the world. By far, the most significant path running has led me to is the New York Road Runners.

I signed up to run the 2010 NYC Half after first experiencing the event in 2008. Times Square shuts down twice a year: New Year's Eve and the NYC Half. You can truly feel the pulse of the city as you stream down Seventh Avenue, enveloped by the digital billboards and thousands of runners on their own missions. I crossed the finish line and immediately experienced the always celebratory welcome of Mary Wittenberg, then president and CEO of NYRR. I didn't realize it then, but that was my second collision with running and a life-altering moment.

Mary and I had been friendly for a few years, and she asked what I was doing professionally and invited me to visit the office and meet some of the team. Thanks to Mary, I was given the opportunity to join New York Road Runners. Since that day, I've worn many hats here at NYRR, and after Mary's departure in 2015, I was fortunate to become its president and CEO.

Not a day goes by that I don't feel enormously lucky that I am a part of our amazing running community and part of a sixty-year-old organization that creates limitless opportunities for life-altering experiences, transformation, memories, and inspiration. I see and hear other people's incredible stories of catalysts for change—what brought them to the various starting lines. I find continuous inspiration from our runners here in New York City, runners from all around the world, and from the kids in our free youth programs to the seniors in our Striders program, and every age and ability in-between.

Inspiration comes in all forms and operates along a two-way street. We inspire others and others inspire us, and that halo effect resonates well beyond the race course. As CEO, I have the amazing opportunity to actually run with the kids who benefit from these free running programs and events for youths. Seeing the smiles on their faces as they hand off the baton during a relay, cross the finish line of a race, or high-five their teammates is just incredible.

A school in Brooklyn, IS 223, has been a significant source of inspiration for me. I was first introduced to the school a few years ago during my weekly youth program school site visits. As I walked into the school, I felt an instant energy, an excitement that came from the kids, the coach, and the principal. They have a great group of diverse kids that have joined the running program with the support of Coach John and the encouragement of the principal. The collective enthusiasm among the kids and the program administrators epitomized the power running can have, especially to young people, and how it can help lift a community.

I've gone back every year to run with the kids and am thrilled to see them participate in our events. They have a few kids who we've sent to summer running camp, and a few who have become Rising NYRR Youth Ambassadors, where they get the opportunity to represent NYRR at events, and they also get help with public speaking and presentation skills. I constantly feel the motivation and dedication of the team at IS 223 throughout my own running.

Participating in all our events and programs pushes me to look for the "new." I continue to explore new running experiences, new distances, new routes, new training groups, and new running partners. I always want to make running an adventure, to tap back into that apprehensive thrill I felt starting out in 1991, and this seemed the best way to do that. Often, you'll find new running opportunities are right in front of us just waiting for us to give them a try.

I'm fortunate to live in New York City, where there is a great running community, offering so many opportunities to find adventure through running. I made the leap into a new distance by taking on my first ultra-marathon at the 60K distance in 2017. Lap after lap of Central Park, I soaked up every ounce of fuel available to me: fuel in the literal sense of water, electrolytes, and bagels, but also fuel in the metaphorical sense of support and encouragement from other runners, staff, and volunteers.

I finished in around seven hours. The time didn't matter to me—I didn't even look at the finish clock. I stayed in the finish area with everyone. We'd all been out there for hours at this point, working together, and I didn't want it to end. I never thought I'd say this, but the 60K was one of the best events I've ever run. It so was fulfilling to bond with others and enjoy the support of colleagues and friends. It was painful, exhilarating, and gratifying—the same way I felt twenty-eight years ago.

I've crossed new terrain within the five boroughs by visiting new Open Run sites, free weekly runs in local neighborhoods led by community volunteers. The program has brought me to new routes in Brooklyn Bridge Park, Cunningham, and Crotona Park to name a few. It has also introduced me to new people coming to the sport at various stages: lifelong runners and first-time walkers.

On Global Running Day in 2015, I met Mauricio Blandino. There's something poetic and even ironic about finding one of my greatest inspirational stories right here in New York City on a day intended to connect runners across the world, share stories, and celebrate what brought you to the sport. It was a perfect running day, and I was in Central Park running and then greeting runners at a pop-up water station to celebrate the day—the first Wednesday in June—and Mauricio was out for a run. We started doing what all runners do when they are not running: talking about running. His inspiring story about how running has helped him in his recovery from brain surgery has been on my mind since the day we met.

Recently, Mauricio wrote an incredibly moving note to me detailing just a fraction

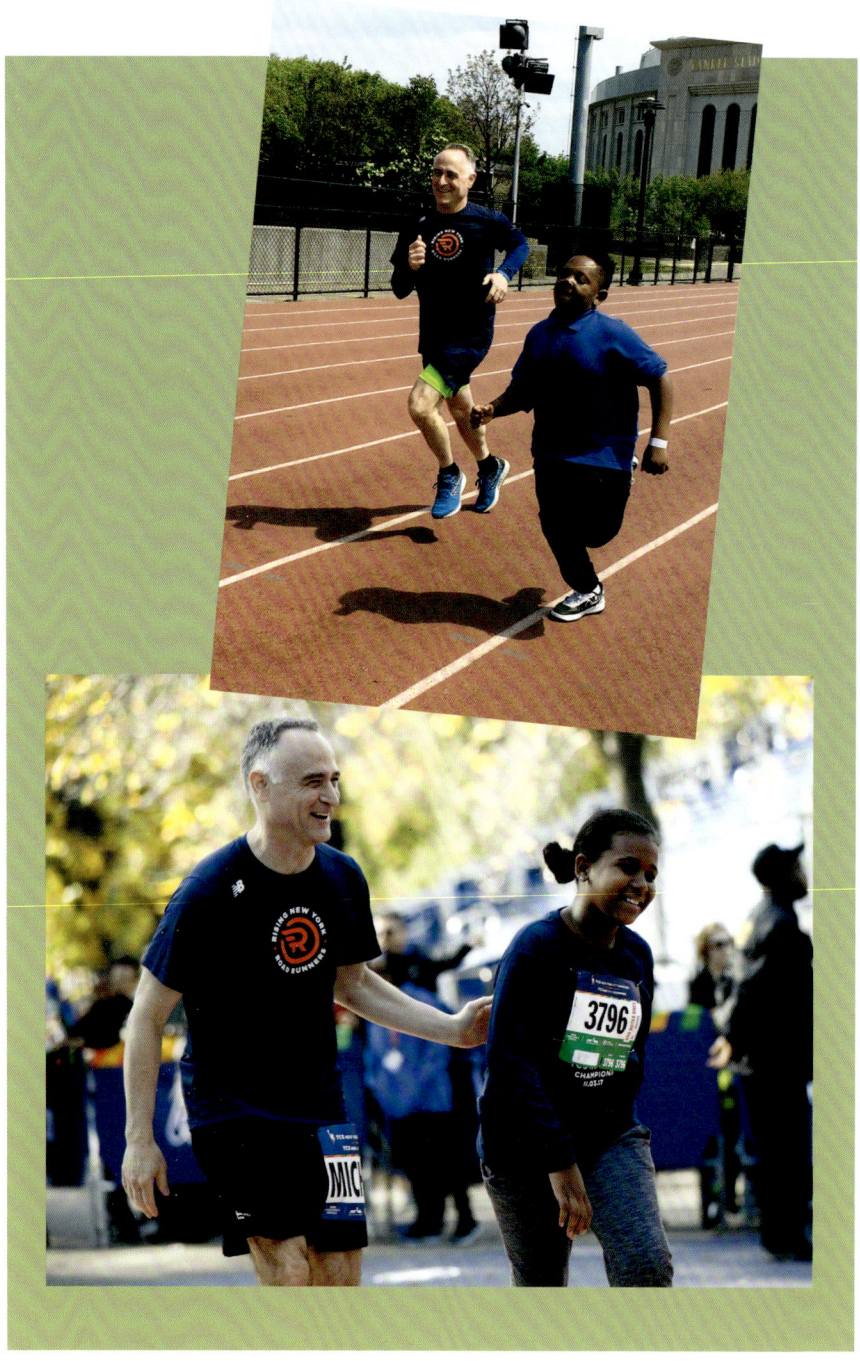

of what he's had to overcome in recent years and the role that running plays in his daily fight. I read this letter often for a reminder of how powerful this sport, this lifestyle, can be. He was kind enough to let me share his story with all of you and continue the halo effect of inspiration:

> "I want to take this time to thank you and the New York Road Runners for the great work you do. Your inclusive organization has introduced running to people of all ages and abilities. I'm one of those runners.
>
> Running found me six years ago, after joining Achilles International after a traumatic brain injury. Walking is what was on the agenda at first. Coordination, balance, vertigo, spasticity, and some visual deficits needed attention, and still do. A year after I relearned the mechanics of running, I attempted my first 5k Race with my two Achilles guides. It was a challenging run/walk technique that led me to my very first race finish line.
>
> I can't believe that from the first steps I took on the Bridle Path in Central Park, I've come to crossing the 2018 New York City Marathon finish line with a remarkable time of 3:45:26 (BQ)!
>
> It's been an exceptional year for me for running, racing, and meeting brilliant people. It has given me a new platform from which I now share my experience with others who are in need of guidance and support.
>
> Running has truly made a new person of me."

"Running has truly made a new person of me." I second that.

As I gear up for my twenty-eighth consecutive NYC Marathon, and twenty-ninth year of running, I take with me these stories of inspiration and continue to pay it forward, investing back in the sport that has given me so much. To borrow a quote from one of my true lifelong inspirations, Bruce Springsteen, and attribute it to running: "You've provided me with purpose, with meaning, and with a great amount of joy."

I do believe I was born to run.

Our paths to running have different origins, unique turns and terrain, and are varying distances, but the community on the other side is welcoming, ever changing, limitless, and always running forward.

Michael Capiraso *has run the New York City Marathon twenty-seven consecutive years and counting with the amazing support of his family and friends. He is president and CEO of the New York Road Runners, the organization that produces the TCS New York City Marathon and the free Rising NYRR Youth Section.*

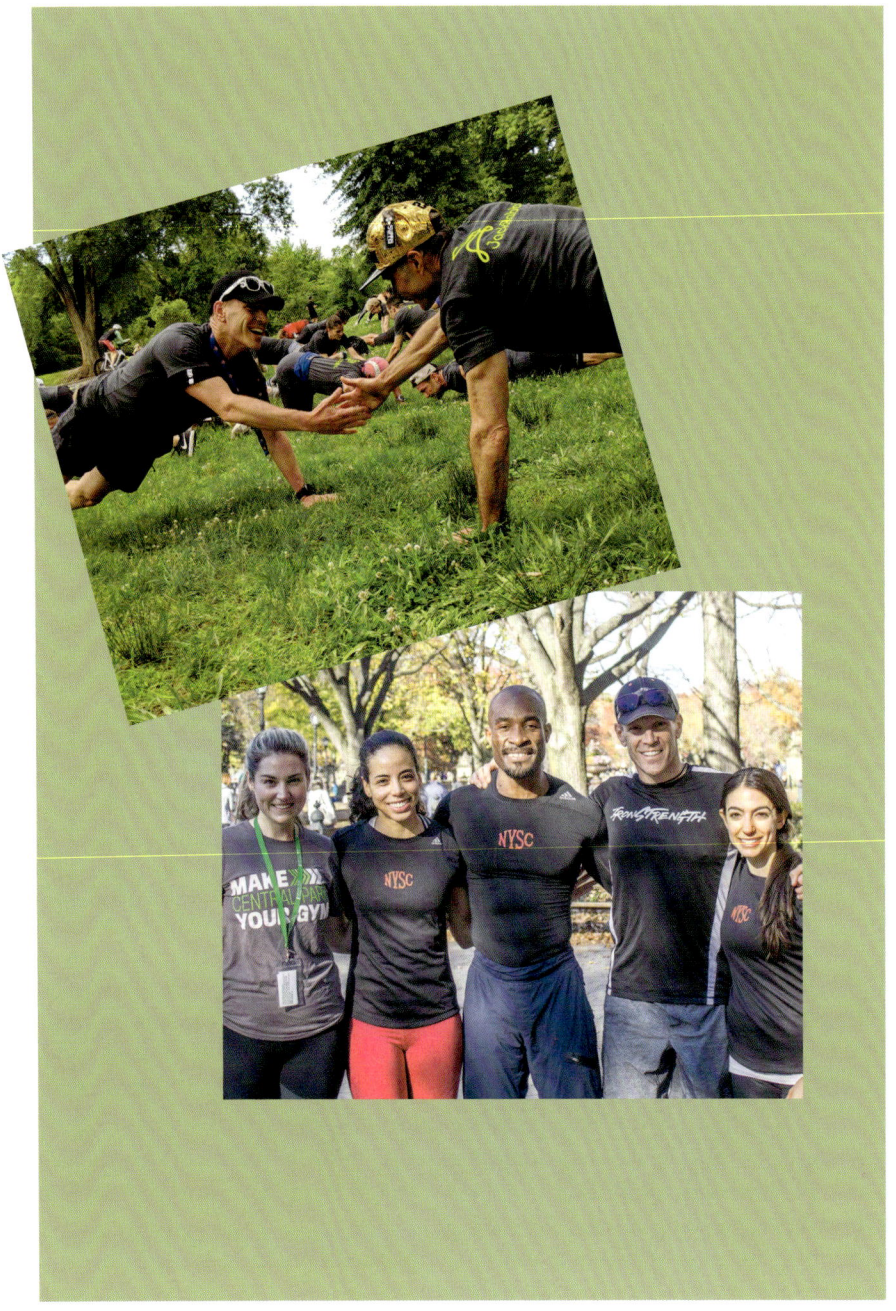

Preface
The Medicine of Running

Jordan D. Metzl, MD

My name is Jordan Metzl, and I'm a runner. I've been running since I was a small child. As far back as I can remember, I've been moving. As a kid, I played soccer, ran around the neighborhood, and biked to the pool. In high school, I played sports and also started jogging. In college and in medical school, movement was a huge part of my ability to concentrate, study, and learn. Today, as a sports medicine physician who cares for thousands of runners each year, I help others stay on the road. In my sports medicine practice, my goal is to keep my patients healthy, moving, and injury-free. I've kept moving, as well, having run thirty-four marathons and many more races of all distances. Running medicine fuels my life and it keeps me going every day.

If one looks at the running culture from afar, the whole thing seems a bit crazy. Humans have evolved as a species to a point where we don't need to run anywhere. Bikes, cars, trains, and airplanes—they're all inventions in the recent past that have negated man's need to run. Advances in technology have made everything, from getting to work to shopping in the store, experiences that can happen from the couch. It used to take a full day to walk twenty-five miles; today this can be driven in twenty minutes. In the future, this will probably take seconds. Does increased efficiency in getting from point A to point B mean we should stop running? On the contrary, it means we need running now more than ever before.

Despite our technological advances over the past few centuries, the human body is the exact same machine it has ever been. We have 206 bones, more than 650 muscles, a four chambered heart, two lungs, and two kidneys. The body was built that way in 1502, and it will still be built that way in 2522.

With diminished activity due to advances in technology, human health unfortunately pays the price. Each year, spending increases on diseases largely attributable to inactivity and poor diet. In the United States, for example, we spend nearly $3 trillion annually on health care. In fact, even calling this health care is a misnomer. We're doing a terrible job of keeping people healthy. Our $3 trillion-dollar bill includes over $100 billion per year spent on diabetes and cardiovascular heart disease, both of which are largely preventable with lifestyle modification. If people moved more, they'd be healthier and they'd cost less.

How do runners fit into this equation?

It's true that runners can be obsessive. They can be selfish in their exercise habits. They can become cranky and irritable when they don't run. They can make minor injuries much worse by refusing to pay attention to the body's cues. I know, I see these issues every day! Despite all of these "runner problems," there is no place I'd rather be than on a run. Seen through the lens of preventive health, runners are saving us money. As has been proven in many population-based studies, runners live longer, healthier, happier, and less medically costly lives than those who don't run. Runners are less likely to need medications, and they're less likely to suffer heart attacks or strokes than non-runners.

More than that, there's something special about the community of runners. In 2012, when hurricane Sandy hit New York the week before the New York City Marathon, the eventual cancellation of the race left thousands of runners from around the world stranded in New York. In our world, a group of fellow runners put together a Facebook group called New York Runners in Support of Staten Island. On Friday evening, we hatched the idea and a Facebook page was launched. On Sunday morning, thirty-six hours later, we had more than three thousand runners from all around the world, dressed in orange, filling several Staten Island Ferries and heading across New York Harbor to help those in need. Our team organized the runners into group of hundreds who fanned out across the storm-ravaged areas. When runners got to an area, they pitched in. Our crew ended up in Midland Beach and included runners from Brazil, England, Scotland, and France, most of whom had never been to the United States. They were all knee-deep in muck, shoveling out houses. Like runners do, it wasn't about complaining; it was about setting a goal and making it happen. The running community is a special group.

Because I am a runner and because I want everyone to run, I spend a good bit of time thinking of how to make running healthy for each person. When I go for my morning run in Central Park, not only do I enjoy my time clearing my head and preparing to start my day, but I also watch other runners. I wonder if the person ahead of me knows that his pronation might cause shin splints, or if the woman with the long stride knows that over-striding exposes her body to a higher risk of injury. I look at all the runners I see through my lens: how can I keep them moving?

If you're reading this story, chances are you're a runner. These are my five tips for staying healthy over the long-haul.

1. Listen to your body. It's estimated that 40 percent of marathon runners will suffer an injury that will cause them to miss time on the road each year. This is a huge number! Some of these injuries, such as twisting an ankle during a trail run or pulling a hamstring during the final stretch of a race, are unavoidable. Things happen when people run. The much bigger category of injuries, called *overuse injuries*, develop over time. The shin splint that turns into a stress fracture, the achy Achilles tendon that develops a partial tear, or the mild case of plantar fasciitis that is disregarded at first and becomes a one-year injury instead of a one-week nuisance. These are all examples of overuse injuries made worse by pushing through the pain.

When I speak to running groups, I explain that the key to healthy running is effective body listening. This means that if pain is changing the way you move, slow down and go see a doctor to figure out what's wrong. This should include getting a proper diagnosis and then a good plan to fix the problem so it doesn't recur.

2. Smile. Let's face it: you're probably not going to win an Olympic medal (sorry to break the news). However, you are going to run until you're ninety-five years old. The science on exercise compliance is quite strong with the correlation between exercise enjoyment and consistency. The more you're smiling, the more you're enjoying what you're doing, and the more likely you are to stick with your program! My advice: figure out what makes you smile and do that thing. Maybe you're a trail runner, or maybe you love doing 10k races. Maybe you're into adventure racing, and maybe you're into indoor running classes. The truth here is that there's not one answer for each runner and the happiness formula changes over time. Pay attention to what makes you smile.

3. There's no one-size-fits-all training program. Everyone comes to the sport of running from a different perspective. Some runners were high school athletes, others spent their time in the library. Some runners have a history of heart disease, others have asthma. Some runners run to lose weight, others are too thin and suffer repeated stress fractures. Some runners are sixteen years old, others are eighty-two. The simple truth here is that there's no single best way to set up a training program because no two runners are the same. Each comes to the sport with a different background and a different history. In my office, I routinely see people who try to follow training plan X, only to end up injured and on the shelf. The basic rule here is that training programs are guidelines, not gospel. If speed training makes your shins hurt, you're probably doing too much. If long runs are causing your knees to ache, you probably need more strength training than your friend who is running the same distances but not having pain. Every runner is different, and every training program needs to reflect this.

4. Almost anyone can run (and they should). From a medical perspective, the medicine of running is fierce. It really doesn't matter if you run a six- or twelve-minute mile; the medical benefits of running reach all aspects of health. Nearly every system of the body benefits from the medicine of movement, from reduced rates of depression and anxiety in the brain, to lower blood pressure values and heart attack risk in the cardiovascular system, to reduced cancer rates in runners versus non-running controls. In short, it doesn't matter how fast you go; everyone should run because it makes them healthier.

5. Think about the race of running longevity: it's a marathon, not a sprint. The final tip to healthy running is perspective. You might have a bad week of running. You're probably slower than you were five years ago. It might get more painful to run as you age. Despite all of these issues, keep going. Running is about consistency, dedication, and the race of longevity. There are no guarantees; Grete Waitz, the nine-time New York City Marathon champion, died of cancer despite a life of exercise and healthy behaviors. What we can say, however, is that running is a great way to create a dedicated, long-term strategy to stay healthy and active.

My best advice? Keep going. Run when you're tired, run when it's cold. Run when you don't really feel like heading out the door, and run when it's easier to sit on the couch. The people you'll meet, the things that you'll see, and the way that you feel—it's all part of what putting one foot in front of the other can add to your life.

Jordan D. Metzl, MD *is a lifelong runner and sports medicine physician at Hospital for Special Surgery in New York City. He has authored five books on the interface between medicine and movement, including* Dr. Jordan Metzl's Running Strong *with* Runner's World *magazine. He created the first physician-led fitness community, IronStrength, which provides workout classes for thousands of people each year. He has run thirty-four marathons and fourteen IRONMAN distance triathlons (and counting).*

Introduction
Ready, Set, Run
Michael Clinton

If you are reading this book, you are probably a runner. You may have never run a race nor have a desire to run one. Runners come in all sorts of flavors.

Or you may live your running life around a race schedule, racking up 10ks, or half marathons, or counting your marathons like many of my collaborators in this book.

If you have never been a runner, you are probably interested in the idea, or you wouldn't be reading this book. Mulling around in your mind are questions such as: How do I get started? What do I do first? Why is it that I even want to go for a run?

It might be that you have family or friends around you who are runners. Or maybe you were walking your dog and saw a runner pass you by and something sparked in you to give it a try.

My friend Linda started to run when she got out of school and was in a new city with a first job. She didn't have time or money to join a club, but getting a pair of shoes and hitting the streets to fit her schedule started her on her running career. To this day, she has an annual goal to run one thousand miles a year. Before she adopted that goal, she would train for a race and then lose her motivation. Now achieving that annual goal gives her a much-needed sense of continuity as she counts her miles, sometimes squeezing in some longer runs as the end of December approaches!

I'm always interested in why someone decided to start running. My friend Ilse is the daughter of a running coach, so it seemed inevitable that she would try it.

A neighbor Yvonne was an established ballet dancer and traded in her pointe shoes for running shoes. "It was painful switching from anaerobic to aerobic, using different muscles," she said, "But I stuck with it, and within six weeks I went from zero to five miles at least six times a week!" Her motivation, helped by years of classical training on the barre every morning, was to keep her physical stamina strong. She ultimately ran races with groups of friends, but today has a regimen of a thirty-four-minute run every Monday through Friday. On Sunday, she'll run a bit longer. She continues to look like the ballerina she was years ago.

What makes a lapsed runner re-engage in the sport, or what makes a lapsed marathoner decide to run another marathon?

After several New York marathons, I had decided I had been there, done that and moved on to becoming an everyday runner. My regimen for thirty years was to run five days a week, usually never more than six miles. I'd sign up for local 10ks and the occasional half marathon and was happy to do that.

My fitness schedule over those years included hiking, tennis, kayaking, cycling, and skiing. I mixed it up and even got swept up in the triathlon craze.

When my sister called to tell me she was going to run a marathon and asked if I would join her, I thought, well, maybe I have one more in me. It might be fun to test myself to see if I could pull it off.

That was eleven marathons ago, with a lot of halfs and 10ks thrown in. I had become a marathoner (again) and realized that it was something that I loved to do, especially the training regimen. I had rediscovered a part of me I had forgotten about.

There are lots of stories of people who quit running altogether or took a hiatus and started up again years later. Although, most runners just recalibrate along the way.

My friend Gambrelle started her running career in college to "get out of the sorority house and have some time to myself," she explained.

She's been running for over twenty years, sometimes with time off to nurse an injury, or with years between a marathon, but always keeping the sport in her life.

If you are just starting out, here are some tips from Jeff Dengate, chief running officer of *Runner's World.*

1) Above all else, have fun and make it a part of your schedule. Don't worry about speed or distance; simply make running a habit. My recommendation is for people to head out for thirty minutes, five days a week. That's just one rerun of *Seinfeld*! Keep the effort easy and conversational. You should be able to talk to a running buddy without being out of breath.

2) Find a running group or friend to run with. Some days it can be very difficult to drag yourself out of bed at an early hour if you are running solo. If there is someone standing out in the cold and dark waiting for you, you won't hit the snooze button. Even better: gather with a group of runners on a Saturday or Sunday morning for an easy jog and a post-run coffee. Check in with a local running store or local club to see where and when groups may meet up.

3) Get a pair of comfortable running shoes. It's tempting to use whatever old shoes you might have around, or to get a pair that's on sale or cheap. But resist that urge. Instead, head to an independent running shop. Don't be intimidated by the expert

staff there, either, because they assist new runners every day. They'll help you find a pair that feels good and meets your budget and needs. Shoes are the one piece of protective equipment you have, and if they are not comfortable, you won't run.

If you think you want to run, it's like anything else: just go out and do it. There is no reason to worry about whether you can do it, because most people can.

Go to the local high school and do one lap around the track. Or ask a running friend to take you out. If you think it will help, hire a running coach to help you find your rhythm. As every expert tells you, start slow. Run at your own pace and don't think about anything more than that. There is no reason you have to run any races or become a world class marathoner like so many contributors in this book. If you get the race bug, go ahead and pursue it, but it should be your individual choice.

My friend Mary likes to say that she is not motivated to do any more races. "I used to do races, but I have enough competition in my life," she told me once as we talked about what running did for her.

What does happen, however, is when someone starts to run, they begin to feel the physical and mental benefits of being outdoors with the wind blowing through their hair. They feel the runner's high, and from that point on, they are hooked.

It's all pretty simple to get started. My recommendation is to spend some time on RunnersWorld.com or buy a subscription, which will include the annual *Definitive Guide to Running Shoes*. As Jeff Dengate suggested, visit a running shop to try on various shoes. My own rule is to have two to three of the same pair of Nike Pegasus shoes I rotate at all times. While many will suggest that a pair of shoes will last up to three hundred miles of running or more, I just look at the soles to determine when I think a pair of shoes should be retired.

For your running gear, keep it simple, but of course make your fashion statement, too. My friend Steve is always decked out in black shorts, top, running socks, and shoes. He is always a well turned out runner! Over time, you can adjust to your own set of accessories from water bottles to Fitbit to other running fashion accessories or gadgets.

Ultimately, you'll have to decide how much you need to wear in the winter months. I've seen runners in long T-shirts and tights running in freezing weather, while the person behind is wearing multiple layers. Figure out what works best for you and your body temperature.

For all runners, it's imperative that you should wear a strong sunscreen, regardless of what time of year you run. My suggestion is to wear a hat at all times, too. I learned this the hard way with too many years of running without SPF or a cap that resulted in skin cancer on my forehead. Today, I'm fanatical about how I protect myself from the sun. And, don't forget the back of your legs and neck when you slather up.

Inevitably, you will deal with injuries and aches, and one of your mainstays should be a roller to work up muscle issues with your legs, hips, or feet. I've been lucky over the years, but the occasional TFL (tensor fasciae latae) muscle pain acts up, which has me on the floor rolling it out or doing squats to strengthen my core. My friend Dr. Jordan Metzl, one of the top sports docs at New York's Hospital for Special Surgery, as well as an author of multiple books on fitness, has some great workouts on YouTube that can help you deal with any set of injuries.

My sister Peg, a personal trainer, has her own virtual training business at www.pardinipersonaltraining.com. This is another great way to stay in shape and deal with running injuries. She offers real-time or on-demand programs based on a runner's goal, including stabilizing muscle exercises to prevent injury or post-rehab work.

Listen to your body as you heal and be smart about how you continue running during the process.

Most everyone will tell you about the importance of stretching before or after a run, although I have to admit that I do very little of it. My fitness trainer, Louis, is a bit appalled I'm not doing more stretching, especially as I get older, and I know that more of it is in my future. I've already started doing it and would recommend that people of all ages do it.

My lack of stretching has become a personal choice based on my own body, and you should determine what works for you as well as create your own training style and technique, your eating habits before or after a run, and your own comfortable pace. Each of us is a unique individual, and you have to find what works best for you. Try different approaches, talk to other runners, test and learn and ultimately, as the saying goes, run your own race!

If you've never run or you are a lapsed runner, I suggest you pick a day, preferably on the weekend when you have more time, and set a time and a place, and get out there and take your first steps. It may lead to years of enjoyment, meeting new friends, and reaching new physical goals that you didn't think were possible. You can start at any age and see where it takes you.

I've always been inspired by Fauja Singh, a British Sikh of Punjabi descent. He rediscovered running at the age of eighty-one and went on to run marathons until he was ninety-two years old, the first one when he was eighty-nine!

So, there is no excuse for anyone. You may not be interested in pursuing a marathon like Fauja, but you can certainly get out there and start your running life.

Ready! Set! Run!

SEE
MICHAEL
RUN

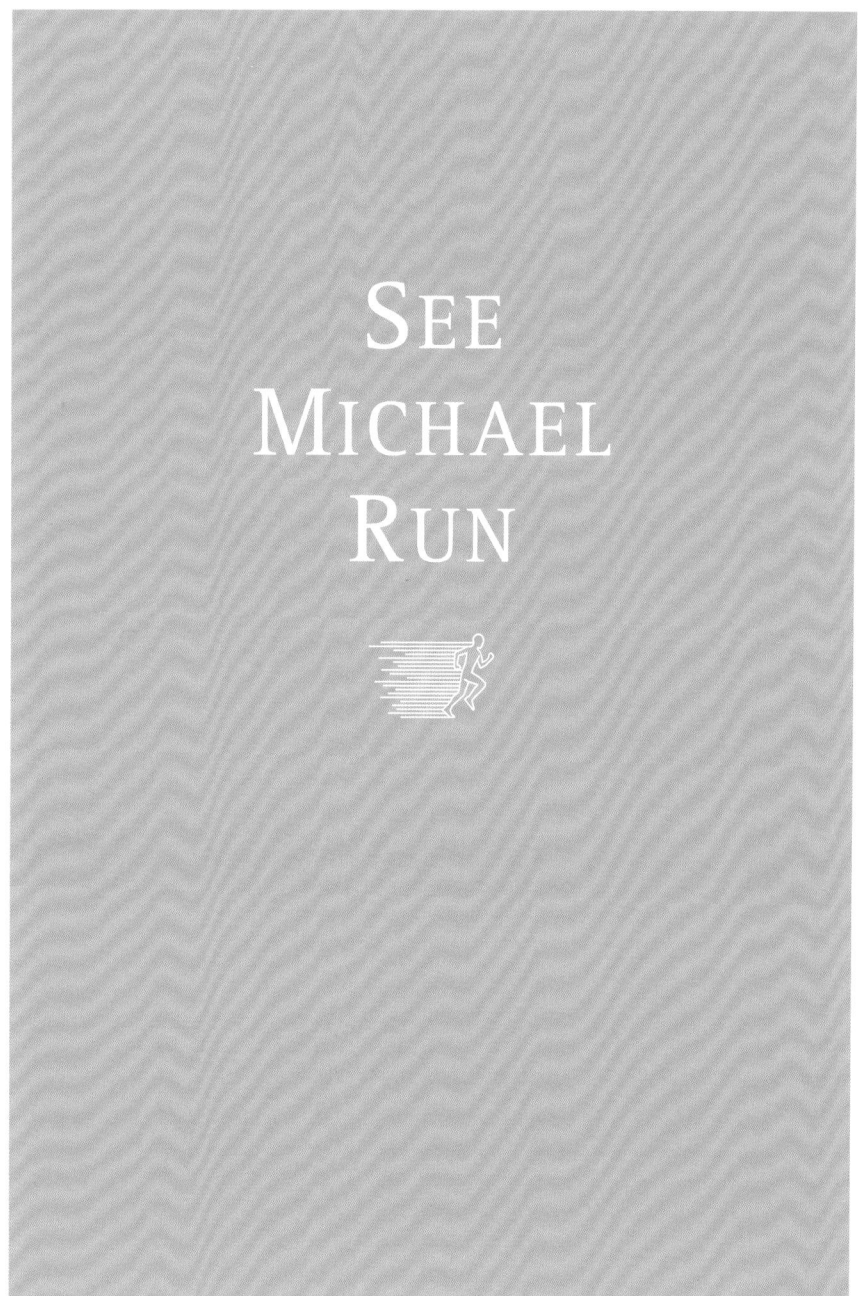

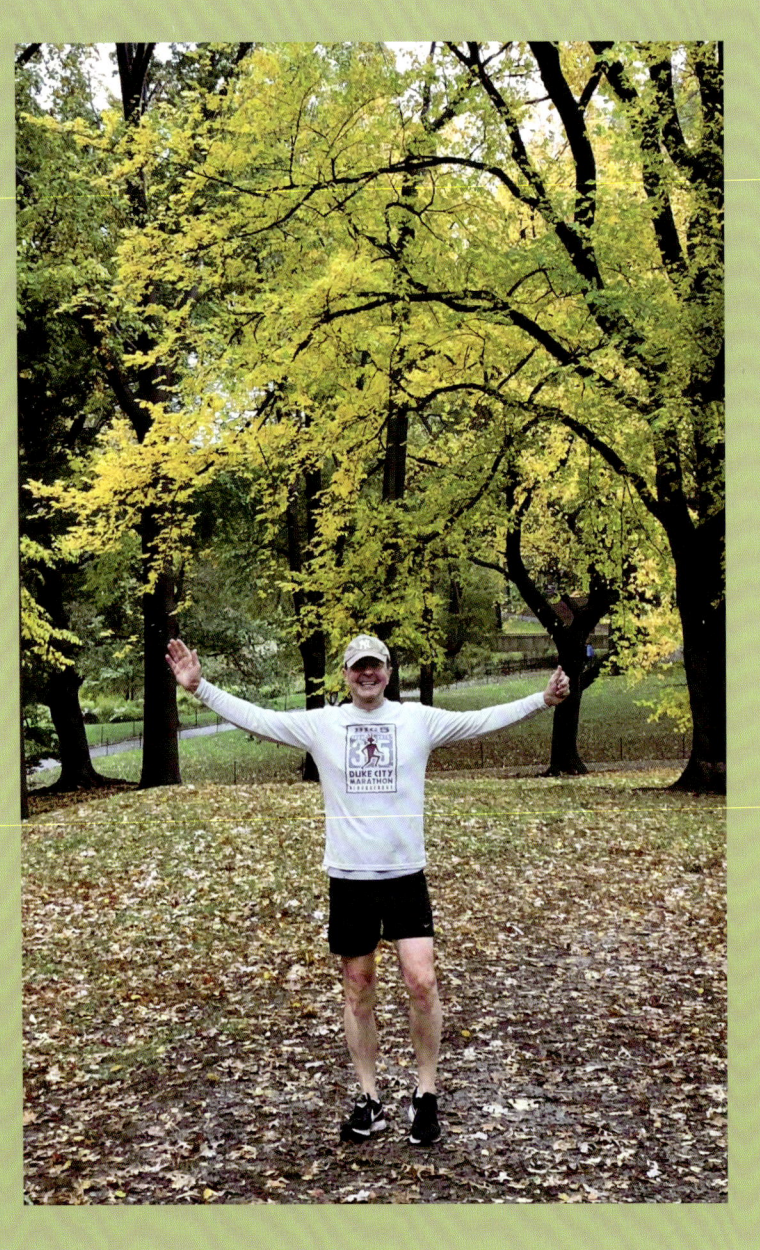

Call Me Runner

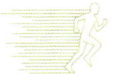 Someone once asked me, "When did you start running? And why did you start running?"

I was in high school, and it was a reaction to something completely unrelated to a desire to pursue track-and-field or cross-country. In fact, running the streets in my neighborhood wasn't even a thing. I don't think I ever saw one person do it! Nor had anyone in my family ever run. The whole idea was a foreign concept.

The beginning was based on the realization that in my city high school in Pittsburgh, the go-to sport was football, and there was no way I was ever going to be able to compete with the big sons of steel mill workers who dominated that sport. I'm not so sure I even had an inherent interest. In the neighborhood, we either shot hoops or played softball or volleyball. My crowd wasn't the football jocks.

I'm not even sure how I heard about the cross-country running team, but somehow it sparked an interest in me and I decided to check it out, as I wanted to participate in some type of sport. The idea of being outside in the park near school, as well as traveling to different places around the city to run, had a curious appeal to me.

The school issued T-shirts and shorts that all seemed too big, a far cry from today's high-tech and sleek running gear. The shoes were also very basic. Nike wasn't even a company yet, and who knows what brand we actually wore in those days. Our coach, also an English teacher, taught us how to move our bodies, how to breathe, and how to develop a stride. All I can remember is that it seemed like a very natural movement for me. It was all pretty basic, unlike the analysis that people go through today to examine how they run so that they can develop their technique.

I was never fast nor did I rack up any championship time, but I enjoyed the feeling of it, and it was the beginning of what would become a lifetime pursuit that brought me both emotional and physical enjoyment. Over time, I saw it as a way to take breaks from college exams or deal with anxiety and stress. But my running was occasional with no real goal in mind.

It wasn't until I moved to New York City that my running life took off. A part of it was a byproduct of being in my early twenties with no money for a lot of extras; all you really needed was a pair of shoes and some gym clothes to be a runner! I began to run different distances, learning that if you could run three, you could run five, and if you could run five, you could run eight. It was just a matter of building up the stamina. Finishing my first six-mile run ever, while my friend Barbara bicycled beside me, seemed like a major breakthrough. We were both astonished that I had actually covered that huge amount of distance!

Running along the East River or in Central Park gave me a firsthand look at my new city and all of its excitement. I made new friends who were also figuring out what their adult lives would be like, and some of them are still friends today. Forty years later, I still love running around New York, as it provides me with a never-ending spectacle of all kinds of people and scenes, a live video in motion. Whether I run up the West Side to the George Washington Bridge, downtown to the tip of the island, or across to Brooklyn, I am never bored.

In fact, running has also become my best way of seeing the world. In traveling to more than 126 countries in my life, I always have my running shoes with me. It has allowed me to run the streets of Stockholm, the parks of Munich, along the Seine in Paris, and more. I've run on the beaches of Mozambique, the hills of Corsica, and the mountains of Mongolia. There are challenges, too. The air quality in Beijing can cut a run short, as can venturing into certain neighborhoods in Cairo or Tunis that might not be safe. Then again, those kinds of neighborhoods exist everywhere. The key is to always have some sense of your course before you head out into the unknown. I tend to ask advice from the locals or try to contact a local running club or running organization when I travel.

I began to run different distances,
learning that if you could run three, you could run five,
and if you could run five, you could run eight.

This is a great way to meet people who love to act as tour guides, too. I've learned about places like Sarajevo and Cape Town by connecting with runners in those towns. But even if you go it alone, seeing a city at street level, through neighborhoods and parks, will give you an appreciation for a place. The sights and smells and sounds are more magnified, and people are inherently friendlier, as they wave and smile as you pass by.

I never set out to become a marathoner; that too happened by chance. As I ran longer miles in New York, I became aware of the running community, as well as the New York Road Runners. Marathoning was just emerging as a phenomenon in those days, and at that time, I was working at a sport magazine and had the opportunity to meet running greats like Frank Shorter, Greta Waitz, and Bill Rodgers. They became my heroes and ultimately inspired me to sign up for my first New York marathon.

Well, the truth is that, in 1978, I ran as a "bandit" in my very first marathon. I didn't have an official number–those days, it was easy to get to the starting line without one, as well as cross the finish line. In total, there were only 9,875 marathoners that year. It was also the year that Grete Waitz set a world record for women and subsequently went on to win nine New York Marathons, becoming a running hero to all of us. The running boom was in full swing, and being a part of it was exhilarating. In those days, there were rudimentary training schedules. A lot of the science behind it hadn't been developed yet, and we didn't eat energy foods or sport drinks. We just, well, went out and ran and drank some water along the way.

I still tease some of my friends who seem to always have a collection of energy bars and jells strapped to their fuel belts, which are filled with sports drinks. God bless, if it works for them. For me, it's still a few sips of water along the way, no food and no energy boosts (which upset my stomach). However, one trick I did learn is to eat boiled potatoes during a long run. They are a great natural energy boost.

I went on to run several New York Marathons (with official numbers) and then didn't run another marathon for thirty years! Throughout those years, I had run countless 10ks and half marathons, but really hadn't been interested in marathoning until my sister Peg challenged me to run her first marathon with her. *I just might have one more in me*, I thought. During that time, I had experimented with triathlons, but the swimming never appealed to me. As I started to focus on the training for the marathon, I fell in love with long-distance running all over again, particularly as I did my fifteen-, eighteen-, and twenty-mile runs.

We chose the London Marathon as our first, one year out from the challenge, because it was my sister's birthday week. The night before the race, we went to a *Runner's World* party and met a man who had run all seven continents, and I was inspired. It spawned a marathon reawakening in me, ultimately leading to running my own seven marathons on seven continents (yes, including Antarctica).

Once I landed on this goal, I challenged my sister to join me, as well. Ultimately, we ran six of these together in Buenos Aires, Kilimanjaro, Toronto, Surfer's Paradise in Australia, and Mongolia (since we wanted to add an adventure race to our list).

The London race was an incredible spectacle of people and celebrations along the route. The city is all decked out to welcome the more than forty thousand runners who descend on the it every spring. Along the route, I was joyous. How had I forgotten how much I loved running a marathon? My sister crossed the finish line and burst into tears of elation. Anyone who has completed their first marathon can relate.

During our travels, we met amazing people from all over the world, but a group that traveled to Antarctica was the most unique. Twelve of the eighty-six runners on that trip completed all seven continents. We were now proud members of a group of fewer than one thousand people who had completed that goal! In my mind, that feat established me as runner extraordinaire! I'll tell some of the stories of my experiences chasing the seven-continents dream, as it will be with me for the rest of my life as one of my best achievements.

When I meet other runners, there's always a spark of connection. We share stories about our races, our injuries, and our goals. Some are hoping to run their first 10k, and others are working on fifty marathons in fifty states. But wherever they are in their running lives, I continue to be inspired by so many of their tales that the idea of compiling many of them into a book came to me (of course, during a long run). Hopefully, you, too, will be inspired by so many of the tales told in this collection of runners' stories, which are also life lessons to be shared, even with non-runners.

In traveling to more than 126 countries in my life, I always have my running shoes with me.

I'm not sure when I started to call myself a runner. It's a part of my identity and is as natural as sleeping or eating. It's a part of my existence, tightly woven into my being. When I'm asked to describe myself, I'll often times say that I'm a long-distance runner. I always get an interesting response like, "Is that what you do for a living?" Some people start to run in high school, but others start when they are in their sixties. The beauty of the sport is that you can start at any time, assuming you are healthy and motivated. All it takes is the curiosity. Ask a friend to join you or just go out on a local trail and meet other runners. Start with a mile, even if you have to walk part of it.

Like many runners, if I go three days without a run, I feel cranky and overweight and unhappy. Even if I'm feeling tired or unmotivated, I know that once I get out there, I'll feel euphoric. It's my natural therapy and way to relax. It helps me make decisions, overcome disappointments, and build dreams for the future. It's also my own connection to spirituality, as I take in the beauty of trees and parks and lakes, always in awe of God's creation.

So, call me Runner. My wish is that I'll be able to do it 'til the end of my days.

What Makes Gambrelle and Vincenzo Run?

What makes Gambrelle run? What makes Vincenzo run? What makes anyone run? It has always intrigued me that some people are just downright passionate about running while others don't understand why anyone would want to run at all. After all, isn't running tedious and painful and doesn't it cause injuries?

So, I set out to ask any runner I could find just what motivates them to run. It wasn't a scientific study by any stretch of the imagination, but rather an anecdotal social survey to see if there are common answers or as many answers as there are people.

My first request was a simple one: just give me one reason you run.

My friend Amir, who has run fifty-five marathons, likes to say "because I can!" His running career took off years ago as a way to cope with a divorce. He has run all over the world, including a marathon in Tehran, Iran, an adventure that he writes about in this book.

Like many people, Chuck runs to give himself mental clarity and to escape from his phone and devices. Running makes him feel younger, especially when he focuses on a younger runner on the trail with the goal to outpace him! "I always finish a run with a short sprint to the finish, even if it's fifty yards out. Sprinting uses a different set of muscles and fast twitch muscles are key as you age," he said.

Like Chuck, the answer that I always give to anyone is: "It's my therapy." It's true that being out on the trails or roads or parks has a way of letting me shed my anxiety, my stress, the issues that I'm dealing with at any given moment.

But that's just me.

Tom ran for the first time when he went on a "jogging date" in the 1970s. It started a lifetime of running that was his impetus to stop smoking, find his carbohydrate burner, and create his own personal temple that he used for praying while running.

On the morning of 9/11, he was running around Central Park's reservoir and found out about the tragedy when he stopped at a local bakery. To this day, when he is rounding the north end of the reservoir, he has a special thought for those lost that day. The longest Tom has ever run is seven miles during a 10k that was improperly measured, and he has no real interest in running any distance beyond that. He has running dreams, where he is running through a leafy park with trails and paths. In the dream, he has boundless energy, his breathing is effortless, and his body feels no pain. In his words, it is a crazy, happy run. Whether in life or in his dreams, running, forty years later, continues to be the mood-enhancer that brings him natural joy and a centering of himself.

Gambrelle has a very special running day once a year. When her Dad passed away from lung cancer in just six short weeks, she wanted to find a way to honor his memory. She and two other friends joined a three-mile run/walk for Strides for Life, a race organized by the Lung Cancer Research Foundation. Ten years later, Team JPS (named after her father's initials) has raised over $75,000 for LCRF. In 2015, Gambrelle became the first woman finisher in the race, a special tribute to her father's life through her running.

Ask any runner what makes them run, and you'll always hear about the obvious physical benefits: a way to stay in shape, to keep weight in check, to build cardiovascular strength. But more often than not, it is also about all the other benefits that running brings to someone's life.

Vincenzo started running when he was nine years old after watching the 1972 Olympics. He said that it helped his self-esteem as a young man and that running "soothes his brain and any fear of life challenges."

He uses running to cope with major disappointments and anger, too. He was running the Boston Marathon the year of the terrorist attack. He had finished the race when he heard the news. He rushed back to the area and covered the event for the Italian presses *La Stampa* and *Milano Finanza*. It was an incredibly emotional day for him, as it was for runners anywhere. That day, he received more than two hundred text messages from people all over the world, inquiring about his safety.

Linda calls it "moving meditation," allowing her to not only clear her head, but giving her time to develop new thoughts and ideas in her personal and professional life. Having thirty minutes or an hour or more with your own thoughts will bring you more meaning than you can imagine.

Spend some time keeping a running journal, not of your actual running days and the times of your runs, but rather the non-physical benefits that it brings you. Did it help you sort out a problem? Confront an issue that was nagging at you? Get to a big decision? Ultimately, you'll find a pattern and you'll realize what it brings to you as an individual.

Running may even help you in a creative endeavor. My friend Chris Richter, an accomplished abstract modern painter who is represented by many galleries from Santa Fe to Corona del Mar, runs for inspiration. When he is running on the beach, he'll stop in his tracks to take pictures of the sea and rocks that he'll use in his studio. On a recent run, he collected several iridescent mussel sea shells that inspired three of his paintings. For him, his nature runs ignite his creativity when he is back in his studio, actually doing the work of a painter.

Every runner has their own unique story to tell about accomplishing their own goals. My friend Jose (nickname Nei) who lives in Sao Paulo, Brazil, only trains indoors on a treadmill four days a week yet has run forty-five marathons outdoors. He prefers to run solo at all times, never connecting with a club or other runners.

Although he is inspired by all of the runners at the start of a race, what he calls "the many stories there," he is happy to focus on his own solo time in the race. He even surprised himself when he came in first of ninety-six runners at the Death Valley Marathon, although time is never his goal, nor is winning a race!

What I've learned when I have talked to my fellow runners, regardless of how many miles they run in any given week, is that there is a common thread: they simply NEED to run. And they don't understand people who don't understand that!

What makes you run? Each of you will have a different answer, but collectively it adds up to the community of runners and how we love our sport.

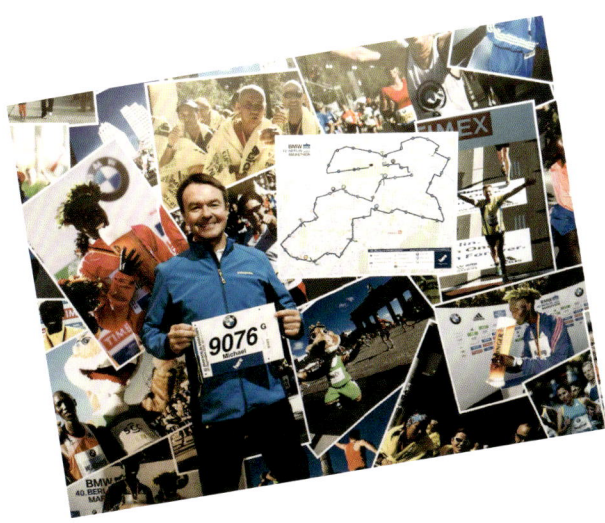

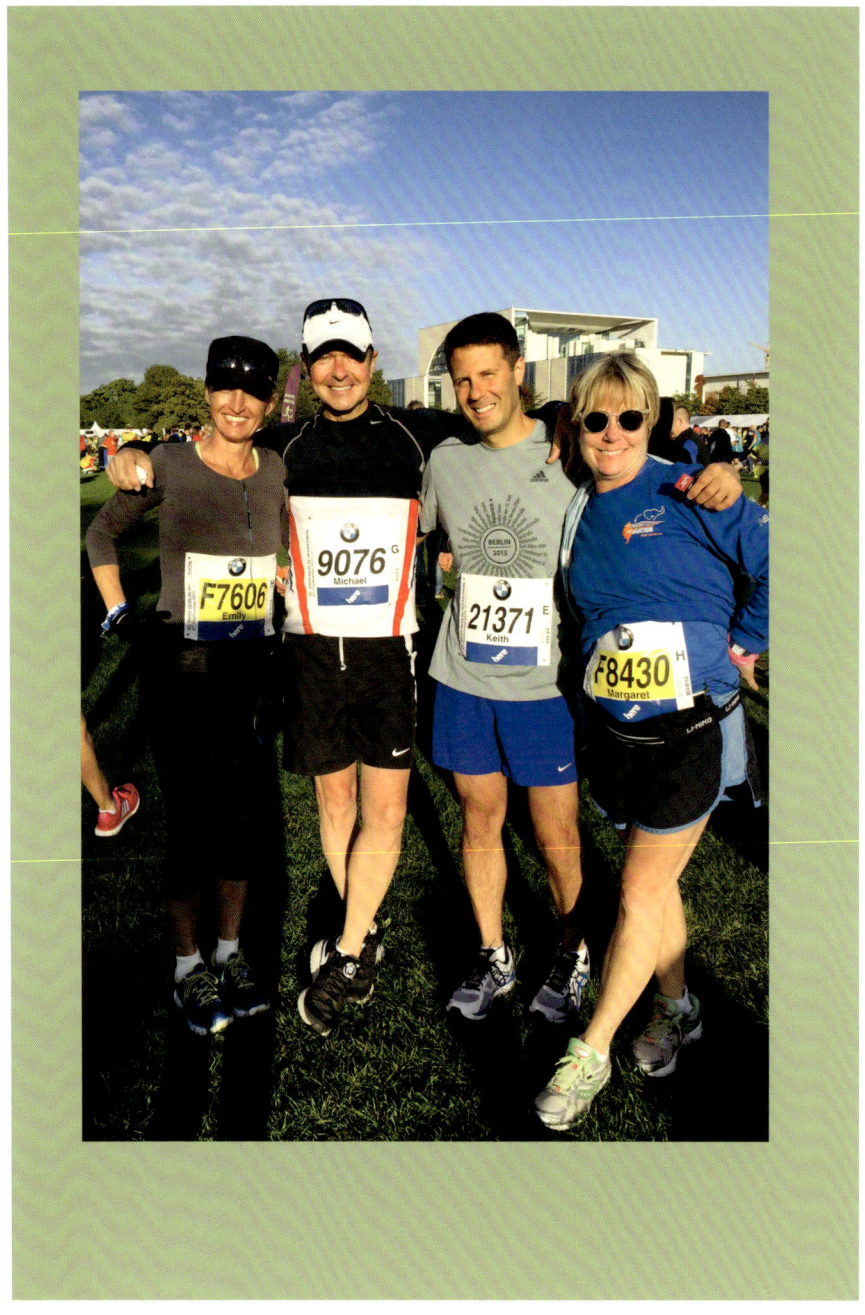

BFF or BRFF
(Best Running Friends Forever)

Most of my strongest relationships seem to have developed through running. Let me say upfront, to my non-running friends, it's not that we don't have a great relationship—it's just that those whom I have run with, well, they are just a bit more special.

Maybe it's the long stretch of time, sans distractions, that allows people to open up more when they are running. I've heard more confessions, secrets, dreams, and disappointments than I could have ever imagined. That could be a book unto itself, but that information all stays on the trails.

A chance run in Central Park led to my meeting Tom, who remains my soulmate, nearly forty years later. Had our mutual friend, Fred, not called to ask me if I wanted to join them for a run in the park, we probably would have never met. We've run thousands of miles together over the years, literally and figuratively, covering every conceivable subject through life's journey.

When I started to visit a new doctor, Keith, a chance conversation about running led us to go out for a run together and today, I call him one of my closest friends.

Keith's goal to run all fifty states has been fun to track, even when I took him off course to run Toronto and Berlin, trying to convince him that seven continents takes a lot less time. A group of us will head to Hawaii in 2020 to cheer him on, as he wraps up his fifty-state goal.

Emily and I became closer as we ran the hills and trails of New Mexico, especially as we talked through how she felt she needed to move on from a divorce that she had been mulling over for a while. It was a painful but necessary decision that would allow her to move forward with her life in a happy and productive way. Our time together running among the aspens, along with her dog ShowLow, has created a bond that I know will last a lifetime.

During her divorce proceedings, I urged her to run longer miles and to think about training for her first marathon. It would allow her to focus on something she could control at a time when a lot was happening. Six months later, she joined a group of us in Toronto as we ran that city's Waterfront Marathon. Cheering her on as she crossed the finish line was a great moment for her and for us.

Cap has been a friend for more than thirty-five years, a friendship sparked by our early running times together, leading to adventure trips around the world from the top of Mount Kilimanjaro to the mountains of Patagonia.

Steve and I have run the trails in Central Park with his dog, Barley, regardless of the season. When my new Vizsla pup, Hannah, reached a year old, she joined the running group, too, discovering the trails and waterfalls in the North Woods of the park. Watching the two run off-leash is always one of my weekend highlights.

> *Maybe it's the long stretch of time, sans distractions, that allows people to open up more when they are running.*

My sister Peg and I developed a whole new relationship as we embarked on our journey of running marathons on many continents. That time together allowed us to learn more about each other, about what we both wanted in our lives, and about issues that we both had to confront.

I'm always on the hunt for new running partners. It just seems that I do better with people once I've had a run with them. It helps establish my relationship with them in unique ways.

My friend Mary would say the same thing: "I've been running with my friend, Julia, for twenty years. We've solved a lot of kid problems, as well as business decisions. Once, I kept complaining about an executive who worked for me. At one point during our run, Julia said, 'You need to fire this person!' She always brings clarity to a situation on our runs." Mary says that running is medicine for the physical needs and talk therapy with a friend for mental needs. According to her, it's the perfect combination for stress reduction. As I grew my publishing career, I was never interested in playing golf, but I was happy to go out for a run with a client or a colleague. Over time, I learned that many others preferred this as their choice of business connection, too.

Early in my career, I was on a team that launched a sport magazine for the active sports industry. Running was a natural way to do business then, including times when I had the honor of running with Adi Dassler, the owner of Adidas, along with other business leaders. A great example was a tough client from whom I seemed unable to secure business. When we both found ourselves in Milan during the same week, I invited him to go out for a morning run in Parco Sempione, one of the city's parks. Not only did we hit it off, but that simple run led to some great business conversations and ultimately a robust business relationship.

I always found that, when running, the playing field was more equal—less one-upmanship as to what your golf score might be and more about finding a pace that worked for both people as we navigated the course. It also took a lot of noise out of the business deals, less machismo. Settling on a pace is the only real issue when running with either a friend or business associate. Sometimes you go faster and sometimes you go slower, depending on your running partner, but ultimately, the competition is the road itself, not each other.

I've done some great business deals over a run, and I've learned that clients are more forthcoming with their goals and objectives. It gets back to the clarity that develops on the course.

It's also a great way to problem-solve. Many times, Kevin, one of my company's publishers, and I would go out for a loop in Central Park to sort out a business issue or two. The goal would be to have an answer before we were back in the office, and we always managed to hit that goal.

Perhaps the best friend or relationship you can develop on the running trails is with yourself. Inevitably, every runner is out there on their own, in all kinds of conditions and usually at different times of the day. It's the time that many of us relish. Ask any busy working mother who's a runner if she enjoys the me-time during her daily run.

"Isn't it lonely out there all by yourself?" a friend once asked me. "On the contrary, I get an enormous amount done," I replied. Another friend asked, "Don't you ever just relax and chill out?" "It's actually how I relax," I replied, which made him even more confused.

Inevitably, every runner is out there on their own, in all kinds of conditions and usually at different times of the day.

Many runners will tell you it's their form of relaxation and meditation. Getting into a Zen state during a long run is about as calming as it gets. When I'm training for a marathon, I prefer to do it by myself, so I can focus on my own pace and spend a lot of time in my head. It has allowed me to have a better understanding of who I am, what I believe in, and what makes me me.

All of that alone time has honed my ability to become more focused. I'll spend an entire run thinking about a particular topic, helping shape my views on life. One such topic was the notion of generosity and how important that is for a person, to be generous of spirit, of time, of helping out in any way you can. Thinking about this subject over many runs led me to realize that I wanted that to be one of ways I'd like to be known and ultimately remembered.

I had to continue to focus on generosity as one of my life's guiding principles. It ultimately even led to a group of us starting a foundation called Circle of Generosity. Our mission is simple: to grant random acts of kindness to individuals and families in need. Without my hours of running, I might not have been able to think through how this could have been created.

Throughout years of running, I've become friends with myself and actually like where this has taken me.

In modern life, we are distracted by so many things that we don't have the time to think, let alone do the work to understand who we are and what we want and need.

Throughout years of running, I've become friends with myself and actually like where this has taken me. It has honed my skills to be direct and honest if something does not feel right to me as well as improved my ability to focus on what is important.

If you're currently in a state of confusion about your life's direction, I say lace up and get out there to spend time with yourself. In the open air, where there is nature and life around you, whether it is in a city, a suburb, or a rural area, you can make the time to get to know yourself better.

And as the poet, Mary Oliver, once stated, "Listen. Are you breathing just a little and calling it a life?"

Breathe deep when you run and be open and honest as you move through the miles. It may give you a new lease on life. And you might even make a new best friend: you.

Time to Run for Your Life

Most runners have an obsession with time. Seconds and minutes in particular. How long did it take me to run that mile? When was I able to do it in less than ten minutes? Nine minutes? Eight minutes? When any of us meet that runner who can do it in six minutes, we are in awe! We clock our runs, our times, our minutes on the trails, and we have moments of pride and disappointment along the way. We wear Fitbits and download apps and pace ourselves with friends, all for the sake of creating our own personal bests.

Yet, for many people, obsession with time and how they use it in their everyday life loses the intensity outside of the runs.

Time itself is one of the great mysteries of life. Philosophers and scientists far smarter than I have studied the phenomena for centuries. Is it endless or finite? Do we measure time in the form of past, present, and future? Is the present all that we really know as a true measurement of time? Stop for a moment and look around you. Focus on your breathing and what you are experiencing in this exact second. Some would say this is all we know is real. The exact moment of the present. Is it living in a real sense or in our consciousness?

Sir Isaac Newton believed that time is absolutely real, while Buddhists believe that time is only a concept that lives in our mind.

We can all debate the essence of it, but the fact is that we construct our lives around it.

We measure ourselves through life events from graduations to marriage to births, along with our achievements in work and personal goals. And we keep a log of our runs with our mileage and our times.

In the practical sense, it is at the core of our existence.

As a runner, if you have an injury, you know that you have to give it time to heal. As a marathoner, you know that you have to put in the time. If you have suffered a loss, you know that time is something that helps you cope with your sadness.

What do you do when you are filling the time that you have when you run?

Are you catching up on new podcasts or music? Do you use it for self-reflection or for sorting out a problem with a friend you're running with? This can be the most constructive time of your day if you channel it in the way that is productive for you.

Since I run a lot, people always ask me if I ever just relax. My answer is that running is my form of relaxing. You don't have to be a couch potato with your face attached to a screen to chill out.

I'm always keeping an eye on the actual time that my run takes, often competing with myself, but what's going on in my brain preoccupies me. I'm either planning a trip or mapping out the next month of my to-do list or working on how I want to get to a long-term goal.

When I was training to become a private pilot, I would review the material during my run to see how much of the information I could retain in my memory. I do the same with speeches or presentations that I have to make, repeating them over and over again during my run. It's also one of the reasons I prefer to run alone—I get a lot of work done!

Time management has always been one of my obsessions. From a young age, I would wonder how much I could get accomplished in a day, a week, a month.

Multitasking has been my way of living, long before it became a word in popular culture.

I'm constantly asking myself: What did I accomplish today? How have I done against my goals? I'll check in on my journal once a month to check the progress I'm making across a wide range of areas. Every year, I create the list of things I want to achieve for that year. It's not that I accomplish all that I set out to do, but the intensity of my commitment to my goals has allowed me to accomplish many of them and made me a more satisfied human being.

> *Since I run a lot, people always ask me*
> *if I ever just relax. My answer is that running*
> *is my form of relaxing.*

The book *The Top Five Regrets of the Dying* by Bronnie Ware has been one of my great reminders that time moves fast and furious, often times like an ocean wave that wipes out what we say we want to do or achieve.

Bronnie was a hospice nurse for decades, working with people spending their last days on Earth. After listening to hundreds of people, she aggregated what she heard into five key themes, such as "I wish I had the courage to live a life true to myself, not the life others expected of me."

What she ascertained is that many people had not fulfilled even half of their dreams and were now realizing that they were about to die.

Life's mantra should be to chase your dreams with a vengeance. What is important to you? Does your family want you to be an accountant, but your true passion is working with animals? Does your partner complain that he or she hates the idea of long flights, but your dream is to go on a safari in Africa?

Do your parents tell you to pick a safe career, but you really want to be an anthropologist? When will you have the courage to stand up for your life before the time is too late?

Too many people argue they are too old to start running, or to go back to school or change careers, yet there are countless stories of people who started running in their sixties, finished college in their seventies, or find an exciting third chapter that has turned their hobby into a business.

Every single day that you ignore the deep dive into the depths of your soul, you are not being true to yourself, and that is what always matters first.

If you have been thinking about running, today is the day to start.

It excites me to hear that someone has made a big decision because they are being true to themselves. A friend of mine groaned when he told me that his daughter was going to pursue an acting career. My response was that if she didn't do it now, she would live with regret for the rest of her life. If she failed at it, at least she would know that she gave it her best shot. It was her time to do what was right for her at this point in her life.

Life is hard work. It leads to tough choices: divorce, telling your spouse you truly don't want children, dropping out of law school to become a journalist. All of them are fraught with unknowns. We cannot predict the future, just the present decision to set us on a course that we believe will get us to who we want to become. And as the saying goes, "Life is not a sprint, but a marathon."

I remember turning down a dream job to be an international advertising director based in Paris. It was an agonizing decision, as I was halfway through a part-time MBA program and felt that I had to see it through. An early morning run helped me sort out the answer, and when I passed on the job offer, I felt relieved, but it was also bittersweet. It turned out to be the right decision; I later received a promotion at work that allowed me to take European business trips at least four times a year. I completed my MBA and moved a lot quicker on my publishing career path.

One of Ware's other discoveries was that people said that they wish they had let themselves be happier. How many times have we heard that happiness is a choice?

Yet, why do so many people continue to live in misery rather than make the changes to find their happiness? A friend of mine is a successful television executive, yet never seems to be happy in his work. *Make a change*, I often encourage him. Find what will give you satisfaction. We all stay in jobs, in relationships, in cities that make us unhappy, yet we find excuses. I'll never find another partner! My company is so good to me. And on and on.

Have you done the work to truly dig into the things that make you happy? A young friend was once deciding if the man she was dating was the one that she wanted to marry. She always seemed hesitant. "When you wake up at two in the morning and your head is clear, what does your gut tell you?" I asked her. She was a new runner, and I suggested that she use her time running to really think it through.

She spent the next month focused on it, ultimately realized he was not the one, and went through the pain of a breakup. Today, she is happily married to the right man and has three beautiful kids. And, oh yeah, she found the running so helpful that she ended up running her first marathon.

We cannot predict the future, just the present decision to set us on a course that we believe will get us to who we want to become.

When I'm asked what makes me happy, one of my immediate responses is running in Central Park! I know this is one of my core go-to happy places. No matter what is packed into my day, from meetings to family obligations, the top priority is to carve out that hour. It's non-negotiable for me. I've made my own list of what makes me happy, and when I flash forward to my own end, I'm hoping that I can say I checked off most of it.

It's okay to be selfish about your own life. But time is running out, so be a maniac about how you use it moving forward.

When I turn on my running app and the voice tells me that I've just hit three miles at a specific pace, I'm reminded that the three miles behind me is over and I only have the three miles ahead of me to complete. It moves fast, and before I know it, I'm finished and on to my day. And that day turns into night and into the next week and then summer comes and goes, as does Christmas, and it feels like it all went very fast. And it did.

What will be your regrets when you are facing your own end? Go out for a long run and have that conversation with yourself. Who are you and what is your purpose?

The clock is ticking.

Running in the Good Air

I know that when you're reading a story about the Buenos Aires Marathon, you don't expect the lead to be about a sports bra, but in this case, it plays an important role.

There was never a doubt that B.A., as it is known, would be the South American marathon that my sister Peg and I would run on our quest to conquer the seven continents.

I had been there for the first time six years earlier and had returned multiple times, as I not only loved the city, but had become the unofficial travel ambassador for all-things Argentina. *Buenos Aires* translates to "Good Air" and so, it's no surprise that it captured me with its sophistication and friendliness of the *porteños*!

My connection to it had also led to me and some friends investing in a vineyard in Mendoza, a small business that continues today with our boutique production of Malbec wine. In Mendoza, we've made great family friends with Cecilia and Martin, the owners of the CAVAS Wine Lodge, a Relais and Chateau which is not to be missed.

Our list of friends there includes winemakers Federico Benegas, Santiago Achaval, Pablo Gimenez Riili, and honorary Argentine Michael Evans, who has lived there for over a dozen years and is one of the founding fathers of the Vines of Mendoza, where our vineyard is located. They are all good air friendships that make Argentina a special place for me.

The country itself is breathtakingly beautiful with vast expanses of land, mountains, lakes, and glaciers to enjoy. From Ushuaia at the tip to Salta in the far north, it is a place that will delight you wherever you go; it's runner's paradise.

Of course, it all started in B.A., a place established by the Europeans mostly from Spain with people from Portugal mixed in during the sixteenth century. From the beginning, this city (and country) has been plagued with some of the most volatile political and economic sagas to hit the Americas. Booms and busts from its early days to independence in 1810 up to the current time.

But the city has always had big ideas for itself, and you can see it in the streets from Grand Boulevards like Avenida de Mayo and Avenida 9 de Julio, both perfect for runners of any level. The city's marathon is the biggest in the southern hemisphere, attracting nearly twelve thousand runners who participate every spring (remember, seasons are reversed there).

The route is a sightseer's dream, as it covers all of the most interesting parts of the city. Started in 1984, the course is flat and a good place for a personal best. We had checked into a small hotel in the Palermo district of the city when my sister realized she had forgotten her sports bra and we essentially put out a bulletin to learn where she could find a replacement, as it was an important part of her running gear.

At the check-in for our numbers, there were no booths that either sold them nor could anyone recommend where she might find one, which seemed a bit odd. Not to worry, we thought, there must be one available somewhere in the city. We went out for a short jog in the late afternoon on the day before the race to find a store.

As we ran through Palermo and other neighborhoods, we stopped at five stores with no luck. There were basic bras and push-ups and sexy ones and ones that your grandmother probably wore, but nada when it came to a sports bra. "What do women in Argentina do?" asked Peg.

From Ushuaia at the tip to Salta in the far north, it is a place that will delight you wherever you go; it's runner's paradise.

After a few more stops that yielded no results, we found ourselves on Florida Street, one of B.A.'s main shopping streets. At one small store, a woman went into a cabinet and on the bottom shelf pulled out a box that had to be the last Reebok sports bra in the whole country. It only took us a few hours and a much longer jog (maybe a five-mile roundtrip) to solve Peg's problem, but now I had a happy sister who was good to go for the race.

That night, we got into a conversation about "good air" and how important it is to surround yourself with positive people who support what you believe in and what you want to do in life. My grandmother had been a major influence in my life, teaching me to always be positive and visualize the kind of life I wanted to live. Our parents had always been supportive; we were told to pursue anything that we wanted to do, as long as we aimed to be the best at it. You can probably easily identify your positive friends and family members and the negative ones.

As a publishing executive, I know the importance of good editing, and that includes people who are the destructive forces in your life. Who are the people who put you down or frown on your big goals? How about friends who are jealous or try to sabotage your ambitions? At what point do you move away from any kind of toxic relationship to focus on the people who have your best interest in mind?

This can include people in your company, too. Stay away from the gossip-seekers and the ones who try to undermine your achievements. Build your alliances and partnerships with peers and those above you who recognize your talents and acknowledge them to you and to others around you. Your own excellence will always prevail the same way your own personal best will prevail when you run your own road race.

The city's marathon is the biggest in the southern hemisphere, attracting nearly twelve thousand runners who participate every spring.

Over the years, I've had many, many clients who have appreciated our joint partnership, and they will always be remembered as the good guys. Frederic is the CEO of one of the largest corporations I've done business with. He always had a keen appreciation for what we brought to him to help his business. His curiosity, intelligence, and friendship are qualities I will always treasure. On the other hand, there are those clients you can never please. The ones who are demanding, always need the win-lose (they win, you lose), and can be downright rude. No names here, but we all have them in our professional lives. They are the ones you have to deal with but keep at arm's length.

As I've told my team over the years, a tough client is a particular hand you are dealt for a moment in time. Learn to navigate it, the way a runner navigates rough terrain. Always respect their position as the customer, but do not stand for abusive or bullying behavior. We had a client, I'll call her Mary, who would send long ranting emails that were often times filled with errors. It made the team crazy. On the other hand, we had a client I'll call Sue. She was collaborative, interested, and always positive. Who do you think got the best work from all of us? Who do you think got the special ideas first?

People who win in business are the ones who have the good air around them. They are the ones that you want to associate with, mentor, help and create partnerships with.

I've been lucky in that my family has always supported me even when some of my ideas seemed wacky. That's when you know who really loves you and cares about you. I've also had to make the painful decision to end long-term friendships that I felt had become too negative, while cultivating those that have been more positive. And I've had to do this with family members, too. There might be people in your family who you cannot move on from, but you can reframe the relationship. How will it work better for you? Have a sit down and explain your point of view. Clear the air and bring in the good air. People always want to be heard, so take the time to listen to the people who matter to you and understand what matters to them. After all, your relationships are more important than anything else.

For runners, being in the present is a constant focus. We are watching where we step, we are looking around us for traffic or other impediments in our course. We concentrate on our stride, our breathing, and our time. We are in the ultimate present moment. Why wouldn't we want this in our relationships, too? Who are the people who are always concerned about you, asking how you are doing, who remember your birthday and who check in on a regular basis?

Many people say you cannot have more than five great friends in your life. Who are your besties? Like training for a race, do you put in the time to nurture those friendships?

My friend Keith, a fellow runner, fits that bill for me. Not only do we check in on each other on a regular basis, but we know what is important in each other's lives. When we're out for a run, we have a list that we check off. Being within the good air of that friendship gives me a bigger spry in my step and makes me feel good that all is well.

At the starting line of the B.A. marathon, I looked around me and realized that, in general, runners support each other. The camaraderie of a starting line is always a special time before a race. During the course, how many times have you supported someone who seemed to be struggling or looked for that support from you? In a race, we all seem to be one, challenging ourselves to the finish, but also feeding off each other's energy along the way.

The B.A. marathon starts in the north part of the city, running through every major neighborhood you'd want to see, including Palermo, Recoleta, the city center, La Boca, and Puerto Madero, among others.

As I ran the course, I watched as runners passed me and also noted when I passed runners. Unless you are an elite attempting to win the race, most runners in a race are happy to pursue their own personal time without an intense amount of competition to beat the people around them.

Have we all learned the lesson that some people are faster than us and some are slower? The natural order of the universe is that this is the case in all aspects of our lives. Someone is more successful and someone is less successful, richer or poorer, and so on. Ultimately, we have to run our own race and determine if we are happy with our own results.

This is what I spent a lot of time thinking about in my Good Air race. Through Puerto Madero Este, a modern city within the city, there is an Ecological Reserve that boasts four lakes and a wide variety of birds and butterflies that live there. When I ran past it, I made a special effort to breathe deep and take in how good my life was at that very moment. After all, I was running a marathon in a beautiful city in another part of the world! We all have the issues that we deal with in life, but we have to also think about all of the great things happening in our lives at this very moment.

During the run, I thought about the people whom I admired most and whom I had learned from. A former boss had taught me that you should speak to a junior assistant the same way you'd speak to a CEO. Everyone deserves respect. My friend Todd always believes in open and honest dialogue. I'm always drawn to people who "tell it like it is."

Your own excellence will always prevail the same way your own personal best will prevail when you run your own road race."

As I thought about all this, I had a great run. There were no aches, no pains, no wall that I hit, I just had a nice stride. It reminded me that when you think about good things, maybe that state of mind has an impact on your race performance, too. This race had been an inventory of all the important people in my life from my family to my friends. They were the group that would give me the oxygen that I needed to not only achieve, but also to get through the rough patches. And I owed them that in return. My approach to life has always been that the glass is half full, that anything is possible if you are positive and focus on the good, work hard and put in the time.

Crossing the finish line at 3:50:53, I thought about how easy this race had felt for me. I was also happy that my sister crossed the finish line, too, despite a shoulder injury and thanks in part to her Argentinian sports bra! She had just completed her second marathon and was ready for the next continent!

I always love lingering around the finish area of a race, watching other runners come in for their finish, some smiling, some in pain, but all elated that they have had a personal milestone to celebrate. The air is particularly good in that space, a time when it's all about accomplishment. If we could only bottle that and always carry it with us, imagine what we might be able to achieve! That's what the Buenos Aires marathon taught me.

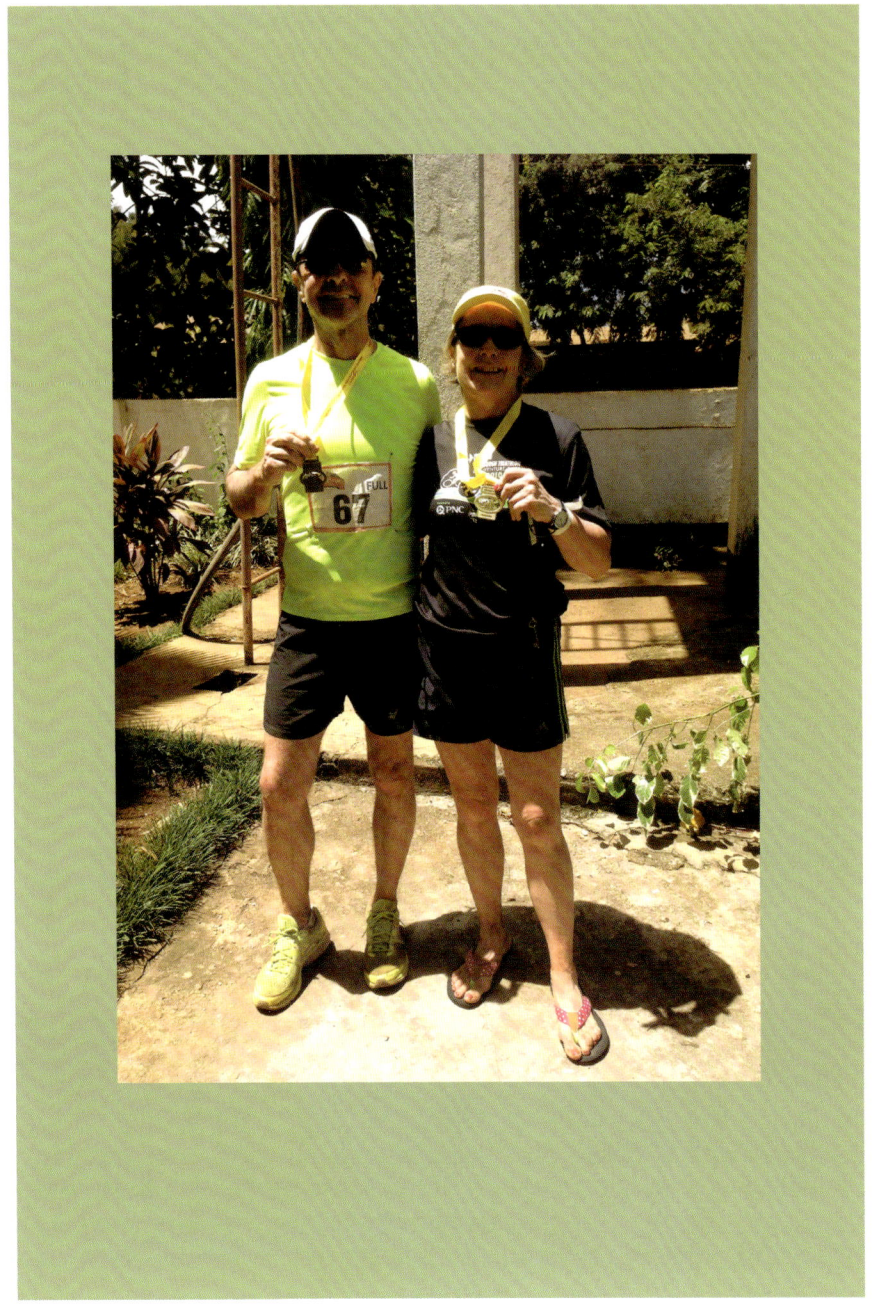

Dealing with the Big D (Disappointment)

Life has many disappointments. Our parents taught us that, as did our teachers and bosses and friends. It is a fact of life that we all have to learn how to deal with things like not getting accepted to the school of our dreams, having our heart broken, or missing out on the promotion we worked so hard for. But we have all learned to take a deep breath and move forward. After all, what is our alternative?

I've always kept a list of my own goals, keeping a personal score of my wins and losses. And, like everyone else, I've had disappointments.

Running is a great way to learn how to manage disappointment because it is a sport that has inherent disappointment built into it.

Ask any runner how many times he or she has been disappointed, and you will get a litany of responses. Injuries that derailed a race, missing a goal time when it was easily achieved in a practice run, having to drop out of a race altogether or just not being able to run a race due to lack of training.

It's constant disappointments when you run, so taking it into stride is a good way to approach it. Using that skill in other parts of your life will make you a better person!

Let me tell you a story from my quest to run seven marathons on seven continents with my sister. For Africa, we picked the Knysna Forest Marathon in South Africa. Knysna is along the Garden Route, one of the most spectacular drives in the world. The town is a great resort destination on the coast. While I had been to South Africa many times, I had not been to that part of the country, so I was excited to have it be part of my run for the African continent. Plus, I love the South African people; they are friendly, fun-loving, and proud of how they're building a new future for their homeland.

It was Peg's first trip to Africa, so we decided to fly direct to Johannesburg and then transfer to Port Elizabeth on the east coast, where we would spend a few days at a local game reserve. From there, we would drive the three hours to Knysna the day before the race to take in the gorgeous scenery.

There was only one problem: the morning we set out, it was cloudy and rainy, leading to a trip with very little visibility in front of us, let along around us. When we arrived in Knysna, the rain had stopped, but it was still a cloudy and windy day. While picking up our numbers, we were assured that the weather forecast was improving and that race day would be just fine. But the day seemed to be getting progressively worse, and as we moved into nightfall, the winds were howling and it was pouring rain.

"This is going to be one miserable race," I said to Peg, "especially since the course will take us into the heart of the forest, which will be very wet!"

Throughout the night, the rains and wind continued, keeping me awake as I obsessed about how I would remain dry beyond the first mile of the run.

> *Running is a great way to learn how to manage disappointment because it is a sport that has inherent disappointment built into it.*

Maybe I would line my shoes with plastic bags and find a large garbage bag I could cut a hole out of to create a makeshift poncho? I thought.

At 5 a.m., we got up and dressed for the race, the rain still pouring down.

As we reached the lobby of the hotel, we found all of our fellow runners looking as unhappy as we felt. A race official entered the hotel and announced to the group: "Sorry, everyone, but the race is being cancelled due to the treacherous weather outside!"

It would be the first time since the beginning of the Knysna Forest Marathon twenty-nine years earlier that the race would be cancelled. The emotion we felt was relief but also disappointment! After all, we had traveled from the States just to run the race, now what would we do?

Every marathoner can relate to the sense of adrenaline and anticipation before a race—we had this pent-up energy inside of us.

"How about a gym? Is there one in the hotel?" I asked.

There wasn't, so we had to rely on our mental efforts to work ourselves down from the physical feelings in our body.

After about an hour of pacing the hotel, talking to other runners, eating a second breakfast and calming myself down, I decided to head back to the room to cope with my disappointment of the day. *Maybe a few hours of sleep will help me,* I thought.

Two hours later, I woke with a pounding headache and stomach pains that put me into a fetal position. I couldn't move and knew something was wrong with me. My sister, who was also asleep, heard me moaning. The only thing I could say was: "I think I need to go to a hospital."

She helped me walk through the lobby, where we learned there was a small clinic a few miles away. As we drove there, I felt progressively worse, wondering what was causing my sickness.

Once I was with the doctor, he informed me that a twenty-four-hour virus was running through the area, and I had caught it. There wasn't much more I could do but rest and ride it out.

As we headed back to the hotel, I realized this might have hit me right in the middle of the marathon, causing me to drop out. "I guess today was not meant to be," I said to Peg. "We'll just have to regroup and come back to Africa to find another race!"

Many people ask me if I had to spend a lot of money to run all seven continents. The short answer is yes, however, it can be done with careful planning and saving. We decided to run one a year over seven years, allowing us to make sure that we budgeted each trip on an annual basis.

Also, I have a lot of frequent flyer miles and that helped save the day with regards to all of our globetrotting. Fortunately, most marathon organizers have access to good hotel rates and side excursions when you arrive in your city of choice. There are also travel organizations that specialize in putting together marathon packages. One of my favorite groups I have used multiple times is Marathon Tours and Travel based in Boston. They make it easy through packages that include all that you need, even your race registration!

Every marathoner can relate to the sense of adrenaline and anticipation before a race—we had this pent-up energy inside of us.

Once we were back in the States, we started our research to figure out when and where we would go in Africa to complete our goal. While there are many great marathons on the continent, including ones in Marrakech, Cape Town, and Nairobi, not to mention the Big Five Marathon, where you can observe Africa's "big five" animals, we settled on the Kilimanjaro Marathon in Moshi, Tanzania.

When I turned forty, a group of us had traveled to Africa to climb Mount Kilimanjaro, so I knew the area and had loved spending time there. I was excited to go back and have a different experience, especially since *Runners World* has recognized it as the number-two "Wonder of the World" marathon.

For ultra-marathoners, Africa also has several amazing races worth considering, including the Two Oceans Marathon, a 56 km ultra; the Comrades Ultra, an 82 km marathon started in 1921; and the Marathon des Sables (Marathon of the Sands), a six-day, 251km ultra held in Southern Morocco, across the Sahara Desert.

An Ultra has never been a goal of mine, although I sure do admire my friends, like Joe Sun, who make it seem so effortless.

We flew from New York to Amsterdam, connecting to a nonstop flight to Arusha, the jump-off point for all-things Kili, arriving three days before the run to an 80-degree temperature at 9 p.m.

From the moment we arrived, we loved everything about the race, which would be a marathon, half marathon and 5k fun run. The overall field was small, fewer than six thousand runners and only five hundred people for the full. While it attracts people from around the world, the field is primarily East African, especially for the three thousand who signed up for the fun run.

While it may have changed since our run in 2013, all of the registration was done by hand. There were no chips nor technology that would be happening along the course. In fact, spotters were at the mileage markers, writing down our numbers to identify that we had reached certain distances.

At the Keys Hotel, the central place for registration, there were no exhibition booths or special displays. Basically, check-in for the marathon was handled at three separate tables.

We fell in love with all the race officials, volunteers, and supporters. Everyone in Moshi was proud of race day in their community.

At our hotel, we met locals and foreigners who were there for the event, and we joined many of them for a beer from the sponsor of the race, Kilimanjaro Lager. Our whole experience felt more like a gathering of friends, as this time we weren't part of the huge crowds that descend on cities for most other runs.

Even though we knew the temperature would be hot, we were happy we wouldn't be disappointed by rain at this race in Africa.

> *From the moment we arrived, we loved everything about the race, which would be a marathon, half marathon and 5k fun run.*

However, the day before the race, an updated weather forecast informed us that it could reach into the nineties on race day.

"Don't run for time," organizers pleaded. "This will not be a personal best. You have to pace yourself and stay hydrated."

"We've gone from rains in South Africa to heat in Tanzania," I said to Peg, "It could be a real impediment for us."

The morning of the race was hot but not unbearable. The temperature hovered around 70 degrees. One exciting part of the Kilimanjaro race is that all the participants gather in Moshi Stadium at 6 a.m. for a 6:30 start.

Moshi's roads are not closed for the race, so as we started, we were dodging cars and vans and motorcycles, along with the occasional goat, cow, and chickens running across the road.

During the first thirteen miles, the heat wasn't too bad, as we all found our pace. We passed local villagers who stood on the roadside but watched more out of curiosity than as spectators who cheered us on.

"Don't run for time," organizers pleaded. "This will not be a personal best. You have to pace yourself and stay hydrated."

We ran past Masai families in full garb, ran through an early Sunday morning market, as women carried baskets of bananas on their head, going about their everyday business.

This isn't so bad, I thought. The course was actually easy and filled with visual delights. There were plenty of stations with bottled water along the way, and the promised heat didn't seem to be happening.

At the half marathon point, however, everything changed. Suddenly, the sun started blazing, the temperature seemed to move up in an instant, the terrain changed to a 40-degree angle and we learned that it would be a five-mile stretch uphill.

During that portion of the run, we all began to feel the heat, and I watched runners around me collapse.

At around fifteen miles, something happened that I had never experienced in a race: each participant stopped running and walked up the long hill in front of us.

Runners sat along the roadside, exhausted, and I thought, *This race is over. It's going to be called off because of the heat and we'll have to come back to Africa a third time!*

Also, I had never walked in a marathon before, and my mind went into overdrive as I realized that my goal of breaking four hours wouldn't happen. The veil of disappointment was enveloping me as the sun pounded down on all of us.

Continuing to walk the course, I looked around and focused on the majestic scenery in front of me. There was Mount Kilimanjaro in the distance. We were in the midst of beautiful coffee plantations with miles of vistas around us, but my real focus was on conserving energy.

At this point, almost as if it had been planned, a group of local kids came out to join us, holding our hands, singing, running alongside us in flip-flops, encouraging us to keep running.

At eighteen miles, we would turn around and do the uphill course in reverse.

It's got to be 90 degrees, I thought. Walk. Run a little. Walk again. *The race isn't called off yet*, I thought, *so I need to persevere.*

Slowly, I got to sixteen miles, then seventeen, and finally to the top of the hill, where I stopped for water and was handed a wet sponge to wipe my forehead. I was drenched from head to toe, my socks sopping wet.

As I stood at the top of the hill, I took a deep breath and looked at the scenery around me.

Walk. Run a little. Walk again. The race isn't called off yet, I thought, so I need to persevere.

"Is the race still on?" I asked one of the volunteers, who looked at me with an expression that said, *Why do you think the race would be cancelled?*

Absorbing my disappointment in my time so far, even though I had no idea what time it actually was, all I could think of was that I only had 8.2 miles to finish.

Starting the downhill run, I began to feel a little rejuvenated. I tried to think about all the oceans and swimming pools that I had been to in my life. Focusing on New York in January seemed like a good idea, too. Anything to take my mind off the heat and a potential forced dropout of the race.

Before I knew it, I was at twenty-three miles, then twenty-four, still dodging cars and people and goats. I stopped for more water, feeling better and beginning to realize that I might cross the finish line after all. My feet were still sopping wet, and I could only imagine what kind of blisters were forming.

At twenty-six miles, there was a turn off the road that led back to the stadium where each runner would take a victory lap in front of a crowd that filled the seats!

Entering the stadium, I was elated that my nagging friend, Disappointment, wouldn't stop my ability to finish the race.

Exhausted, I crossed the finish at 4:29, only thirty minutes or so off my desired time. I hobbled over to the hospitality tent, where I downed three bottles of water and three beers and poured another three bottles of water over my head and body.

At the end of the day, we learned that of the 500 runners, only 238 finished the race. Surprisingly, I had placed 139th, realizing that all is relative and that I was no longer disappointed, but rather proud and happy.

Peg also finished the race and had been a lot smarter than me. When the heat hit hard, she made the right decision to turn the race into a fun run. She stopped and

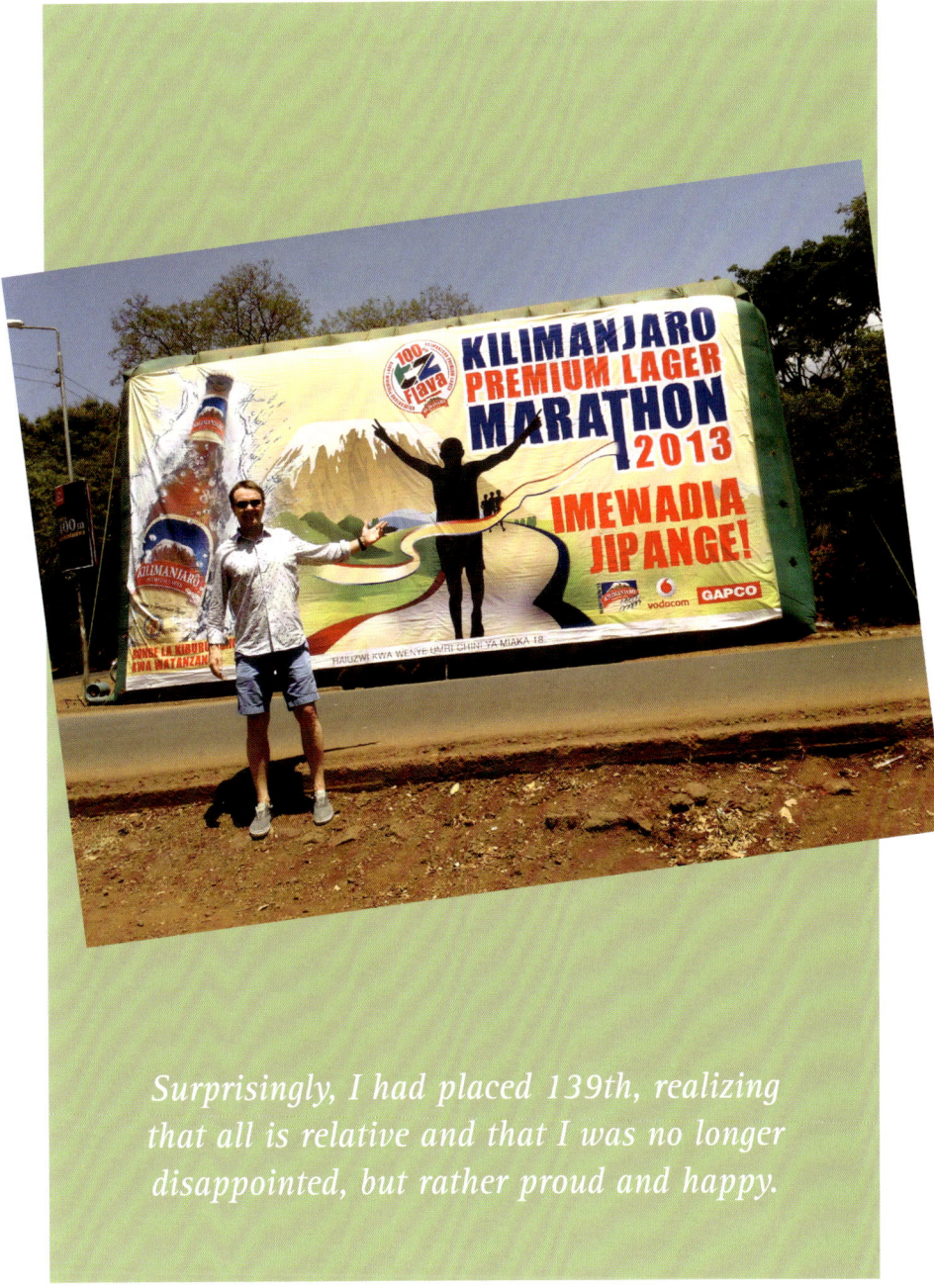

Surprisingly, I had placed 139th, realizing that all is relative and that I was no longer disappointed, but rather proud and happy.

danced to the local bands, who played along the way, she chatted with volunteers at the water stations, and when she walked, she focused on the beauty of Africa around her.

She had done the right thing and followed the advice of the organizers. Forget about time. Just go out there and enjoy the race. My sister taught me a great lesson that day.

Throughout my running career, disappointment has taken many forms for me. With a hip flexor injury, I had to downgrade from a marathon to a half marathon in Albuquerque. Planning a run in Oslo had to be abandoned due to a heavy business schedule, not to mention nursing injuries during the training.

In 2012, after nearly thirty years, I had decided to run my hometown race again, the New York Marathon. I was excited about the prospect and asked my mother to bring Nicolas, my great nephew, to New York so he could have the experience of going to the Javits Center to witness the exhibition festivities and cheer on his uncle during the race. At ten years old, I thought it might give him some inspiration to think about running in his future.

The week before the race, Hurricane Sandy hit the East Coast, devastating many parts of New Jersey and New York City neighborhoods along the Atlantic Ocean. Staten Island, where the marathon starts, had been hit hard.

By Wednesday of that week, the race was still on, as tens of thousands of visiting runners began to descend on New York. By Thursday night, preparations for the Sunday race continued to expand, however the true damage done to parts of the city emerged on the local news.

Many runners made attempts to raise funds for the victims and started thinking of grassroot efforts to help the local neighborhoods.

On Friday, the public, the media, and even some of the runners called for the race to be cancelled. Late Friday, for the first time in its forty-two-year history, the decision was made to cancel the race.

I had gotten home from work to find my nephew playing a computer game. When he looked up, he said, "Uncle Michael, the marathon has been cancelled!"

"Ha," I said, "don't tease me like that."

"It was just on the news," he said.

Turning up the television, sure enough, I saw the mayor and the New York Road Runners president make the announcement.

Like many runners that day, I still hadn't realized the full impact that Sandy had had on our city. As the details were released, it became apparent that cancelling the race was the right decision. We had to concentrate on the victims of the storm and figure out how we might help.

I called my friend, Lucy, who at the time was the editor of *SELF* magazine, to ask her if she knew of any efforts that runners were making to help out.

Around the city, running groups were forming to volunteer their time, and our mutual friend Dr. Jordan Metzl was asking runners to join the group named New York Runners in Support of Staten Island.

On Sunday morning, the day of the cancelled race, thousands of runners traveled to Staten Island to help the devastated neighborhoods. Metzl's group all dressed in orange and met at the ferry with backpacks full of clothes and everyday household goods. When we crossed over to the island, we ran four miles in small groups to deliver our goods to makeshift shelters to help the needy.

Forget about time. Just go out there and enjoy the race. My sister taught me a great lesson that day.

When we ran four miles back to the ferry, all of us felt great pride that we had done something with our running skills, channeling our pent-up marathon need in a productive way that gave back to our fellow New Yorkers.

For many of the marathoners that year, it was a great disappointment, especially for the first-timers. But it was only a race, and there will always be races to be run.

The organizers of the Philadelphia Marathon extended entries to people who had planned to run New York. and I ended up running Philly that year. Maybe it was good karma for the work we all did on Staten Island, as I had one of my better times at 3:52 for that race.

But more importantly, it was a great lesson for young Nicolas: what could have been an expression of disappointment became an action to help other people.

When we explained to him that that was what was more important, he understood.

Runners will always have disappointments, but it's what we learn from them and how we channel them that provides the life lesson.

Injuries will heal, times will improve (or not), but we all learn to regroup and find another run.

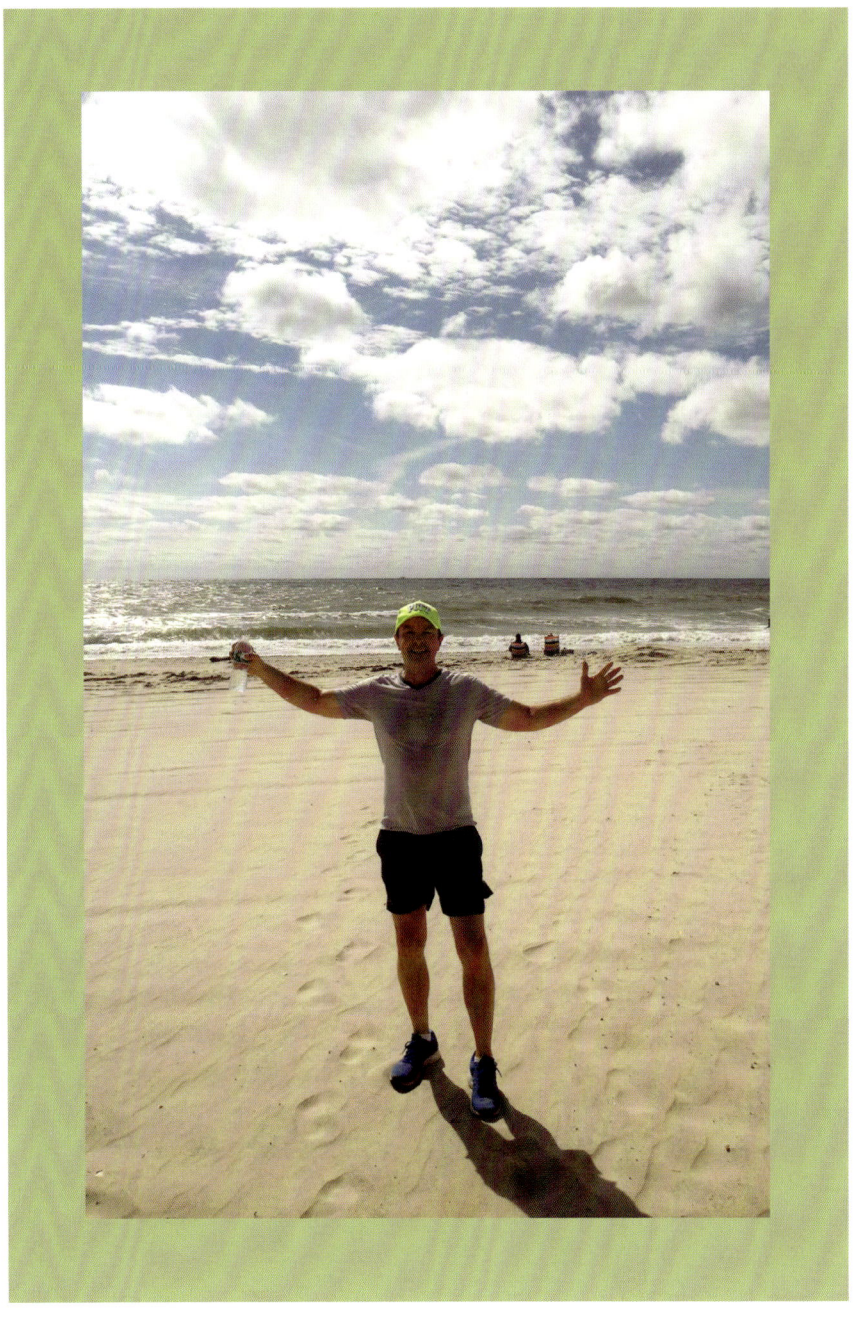

The 3-Day Roundtrip to an Australian Marathon

Whenever Americans talk about Australia, inevitably the subject of time comes up. It's twenty-four hours door to door from New York City to Sydney. Australia is fourteen hours ahead of New York, but you cross the International Dateline and lose a day when you fly there.

When you fly back to the West Coast, you actually arrive earlier than when you left (picking up the day on the way home). The Los Angeles to Sydney flight is one of the longest in the world.

Yup, let's just put it out there: this is one faraway place for Americans. But it's faraway for most people in the world. Even from Hong Kong, one of the closest capitals, the flight is ten hours. However, Australians take this all in stride. They hop onto a ten-hour flight the way New Yorkers fly to Florida.

I had been to Australia four times, and I have gone in coach, business class, first class, and on a G5 for a business trip. Trust me, the G5 wins for best way to get there. For my fifth trip, sister Peg and I were heading to the Gold Coast on the continent's east coast to add our fourth continent in the quest of running all seven continents. The big discussion was how much time we should give ourselves to for a time adjustment before race day.

Due to busy schedules, we settled on two days, which in hindsight was a bit ridiculous. We'd take the nonstop QANTAS flight from Los Angeles to Brisbane, then drive the one hour to the Gold Coast. The flight would land at 6 a.m. and we would run forty-eight hours later.

We'd have to use the forty-eight hours wisely, as this kind of jet lag can be brutal. And to add to the story, I had been nursing a head and chest cold, not to mention an ankle injury that happened on one of my eighteen-mile training runs.

But we had it all laid out. It would be about relaxing: a few naps, a light two-mile jog, early to bed with half a sleeping pill to guarantee a good night's sleep on night one. We even caught a movie and woke up on race day feeling pretty good.

Trying to time one's body clock is a very individual thing, and I pride myself on knowing what works best for me. After years of globetrotting, I had challenged myself to some pretty brutal schedules. Let's call it marathon traveling! When I finished the Buenos Aires marathon, several hours later I boarded a flight to Paris and then changed planes to London to make it in time for a major company event taking place that evening. In the past, I had flown to Paris for a meeting and turned around and flew home the same day. It wasn't unusual for me to come home from places as exotic as Nepal, Myanmar, or India and go to work the next day, or in the case of a trip home from South Africa, actually go home, shower, and go to the office. Time zone resiliency just seemed part of my skillset. Although landing somewhere and running a marathon added a whole different challenge.

> *Trying to time one's body clock is a very individual thing, and I pride myself on knowing what works best for me.*

I love Australia. And I love Australians. I met my first group of them when I was an eighteen-year-old backpacking in Europe. The famous "gap year" for young Australians is a way for them to go around the world for a year, as they may not have the opportunity in the future. I've loved hearing stories from my friend Jenny's son, Kim, who took the Trans-Siberian, traveled all over America, even snagging tickets to the Super Bowl, before moving on to South America.

Australians have that can-do, optimistic, sunny disposition that I'm drawn to, not to mention they are friendly, athletic, and seem to glisten in the Southern Hemisphere sun. Is it my imagination, or does everyone look like they stepped out of a Quiksilver ad? Okay, there are fat and out of shape Australians, too, but I'm stuck on my own image of them!

The Gold Coast is a forty-mile stretch of beach towns including Surfer's Paradise, Broadbeach, Palm Beach, and Currumbin, to name a few. In many ways, it reminds me of the Florida Coast with some low-rise buildings followed by high-rise gleaming condos and apartments. Q1, the tallest building in the country, is here and is also one of the highest residential buildings in the world. So, don't picture small beach towns; picture glistening, developed high-rises with lots of shops, restaurants, and clubs. This is where many Australians come to enjoy the surf and sand. One of our favorite moments was the thirty-minute drive south to Currumbin, where we went to a local surf club built on Elephant's Rock. We sat and had breakfast, watching the sea, and looked north to Surfer's Paradise and Broadbeach, as an Oz-like apparition in the distance.

This was my first time in this part of Australia. Past trips had been to Sydney,

Melbourne, the Great Barrier Reef, Tasmania (to hike in the rainforest), and Thredbo (to hike the tallest mountain in the country). More on all of that in a moment.

The history of Australia is well-known: a penal colony established in the 1830s, as Brits and Scots and Irishmen were sent to this desolate place at the end of the world. At the same time, America was already sixty years into its own independence, and in France, Victor Hugo and Delacroix were busy creating works of genius. In Australia, they were hunting kangaroos.

Race morning arrived and, like most of Australia, this group is organized: shuttle buses that run along the main road to the starting gate; lots of portable restrooms without long lines; booths with food, water, and coffee. Race time was 7:10 a.m. with 5,086 registered marathoners. We had done our carb loading and felt good to go.

The start was in a beautiful park alongside the ocean, and the early sun began to rise amid just the right amount of cloud coverage to assure a somewhat cool run. The head cold was still there and the ankle was a little sore, but overall, I felt well-rested and ready to go. Most of the runners were from Australia and New Zealand, although I saw a few Japanese contingents and, like most marathons, the starting line is filled with a bit of anxiety and a bit of "let's get this run going" mentality.

BANG. The starting gun, and we're off . . . along a gorgeous course that straddles the ocean as the early morning sunrise turns the sky into beautiful hues of pinks and purples. I was tracking well, feeling good, hoping to do the first 10k to get my rhythm and my pace in place. At 10k, I planned to do a cross-check on my body parts and set my pace. Along the way, we passed ample water stations, and many surfers with boards waiting to get across our group to hit the early morning waves.

We sat and had breakfast, watching the sea, and looked north to Surfer's Paradise and Broadbeach, as an Oz-like apparition in the distance.

At 10k, I was good and ready to work to 15k, but in that stretch, my ankle began to feel a little funky. So, I took my mind off of it—*quick, can you name ten famous Australians?* I ask myself, and for some reason, Nevil Shute enters my mind! Why an Australian who wrote a book more than fifty years ago came to mind first, don't ask! Maybe I was channeling the title On the Beach . . . Then came Olivia Newton John (now that's a juxtaposition). Mel Gibson. Nicole Kidman. Rod Laver. Russell Crowe. Dame Joan Sutherland. Keith Urban. Colleen McCollough. Ian Thorpe. An eclectic group for sure. There are some music groups, too. Aren't the Bee Gees Australian? Air

Supply. INXS. AC/DC. How about the Wiggles? The game helped me not think about the nagging ankle.

At 15k, I found the official pace runner for the four-hour marathon, and he was leading a pack of around twenty runners. And since four hours was my goal, I jumped in. I usually don't travel in packs, but this guy was great. A young Japanese Australian, he was a great motivator, and I forgot my ankle and moved right into the pace. I was in heaven. Every runner finds their pace at some point, and I had caught my stride. I love long distance running and the people who do it. We all appreciate what running does for our minds, bodies, and souls and running with other marathoners always makes me feel like I'm home. I was a part of the pack and we moved as one.

All was good until around 30k, when my ankle injury sent a pain up my leg that sent me for a loop. I take it in stride, until I realize that, at around 31k, I needed to stop and stretch it out. I jumped out of the pack, miserable that I couldn't be with them anymore. I hoped I'd catch up, but in listening to my body, this pain was not good. And I worried about how bad it could get.

At 31k, I stretched out my legs and my hip flexors, but it didn't do much good. Plus, I felt some congestion from my cold, but I decided to carry on, my four-hour pace runner way off into the distance. I had done the London race in 4:08 and Buenos Aires in 3.50, and I was setting a goal of breaking four hours again, but now that didn't seem possible. With another 11.2k to go, I wondered if I could even finish, but I started up again. Who are the other famous Australians? Cate Blanchett, Hugh Jackman, Peter Allen, Evonne Goolagong . . .

From 31k to 36k, I was dealing with pain up my entire right leg. Damn. I should have done more icing of my ankle. The sun began to shine and it was getting hotter. Drink some water. Ignore the pain. And then at 36k, I hit it—the famous wall. No, I slammed into it. Usually, I could manage my way through it, but for some reason, this time it wasn't working for me. *Two days was not enough to adjust to the time difference,* I thought. I was wiped out.

I lost my pace, and with the heat and my leg pain, I even felt a little delirious. I had never felt this way in any of my past marathons. This wasn't good, and then I ran out of other famous Australians. I was coming up empty.

One of the great reasons to go to Australia is for the adventure of it. And while I haven't done the outback yet, I have had some great adventures here. We went to Thredbo to hike to the top of Mount Kosciusko, the tallest mountain on the continent, and we've snorkeled on the Great Barrier Reef. But one of the most memorable was a trip to Tasmania off the Southern Coast.

Flying into Launceston, we went there specifically to hike Cradle Mountain, one of the great rainforests in this part of the world. And it didn't disappoint us. In fact, the hikes were magnificent, with views of the low-hanging canopies and the mist over the trees and bushes. But it was the leeches that really added to the excitement.

About two hours into the hike, our guide casually mentioned we might want to look at our hiking boots, and several of us looked down to find our shoelaces covered with leeches. But it wasn't until we opened our ponchos, when we found twenty or thirty leeches all over our legs, that we all looked at each other and didn't know whether to laugh or yell. As it turned out, we did a little of each until the guide informed us in a very calm voice that it wasn't possible to hike in the rainforest without this happening.

Why didn't he tell us beforehand? "Well, a lot of people opt out of the hikes," he said. Well, yeah, I get it.

I lost my pace, and with the heat and my leg pain, I even felt a little delirious.

The fact is that leeches can't really hurt you; it's just the idea of them. Or so we thought, until our guide told us the story of someone who had a leech crawl into their eye and behind their eyeball. *Nice*, we thought, as we looked at each other to make sure there were no leeches on our faces, or anywhere near our eyes, nose, or ears!!

To sit and pick the leeches off seemed pointless, as more would come, so we carried on with the hike. But when we finished, one of the first things we did was strip down to find, yes, more leeches inside our clothes. I'll spare you the details, but just imagine the next forty minutes: pulling leeches off our legs and arms and stomachs, and well, you get the drift.

And while leeches are harmless, it does make a great story, don't you think?

At 36k, I wished my only problem was leeches. But sometimes you just have to reach inside of yourself to find that secret reservoir that we all stash away for the right occasion. Most people will tell you that while you can feel pain running a marathon, it's a head game, and I decided that I had to find the inner resolve to keep moving forward.

My pace was slower and I was climbing over the wall. And I decided to do what marathoners do: step out of my own body. Transcend the physical. Get into a Zen state. And that's exactly what I did from 36k to 39k. And as I moved past the 39k mark, the crowds began to swell, and I transferred myself to them, drawing in their energy.

I looked at the crowds and my fellow runners. Running alongside a young woman, I asked her, "How are you feeling?" With tears in her eyes, she looked at me and said, "I can't make it, I'm stopping, I'm too tired." Well that did it for me—a rush of adrenaline hit me. We were 3.2k away from the finish line; I said to her, "You aren't quitting, and we're going in together." And that's exactly what we did.

4:11:48.

I didn't break my four-hour goal, but my young Aussie friend and I made it and gave each other a smile and a hug as we limped away together to the recovery area. We didn't even exchange names, but we had helped each other in one of life's tough moments.

Flying to Australia to run a marathon two days later with a cold and an injury wasn't the smartest thing I've ever done, but it made me think about all of the exotic marathons in the world in far-off destinations, especially since I knew that Antarctica would be my last and final continent.

While the Gold Coast was a pretty easy course, my own self-imposed conditions led me to think that I wanted to push myself in future runs. Maybe I'd travel a bit further to find more obscure runs that would push me to new limits.

I had already decided I didn't want a typical city run for my Asia continent. Everyone talked about the Great Wall of China Marathon as one of the most grueling, but I still wanted something different. For the intrepid marathoner, there are lots of races to choose from. The Baikal Ice Marathon in Russia is on ice. There is the North Pole Marathon, one of the most expensive runs to enter, and the Everest Base Camp Marathon, which includes a hike to the Everest Base Camp and then a 26.2-mile run. That one appealed to me the most but would require a significant amount of time to acclimatize and complete the run.

While I had struggled through the Gold Coast race, I was ready for the next level. Peg finished a bit after me and she, too, was exhausted. We learned that her husband, Bob, and son Bobby were able to watch her cross the finish line via a live video broadcast on the marathon website.

We both suffered through our pain together, supporting each other. We showered and prepared to leave for the airport to fly to Sydney. We slept very well that night after celebrating with some friends.

The next morning, as we walked along Circular Quay, a runner passed us. We looked at each other and Peg said, "Don't you feel like a little run?"

That night, we flew home after our three-day trip to Australia, our fourth continent under our belt. We had learned that we could push ourselves more than we thought possible and agreed that this was the life lesson we would take home from down under.

Business Decisions (On the Run)

Subject Line: I just went out for a run!

Many of my colleagues know this familiar email subject line when it appears on their screens. It usually means that I've come up with a slew of ideas, some good, some bad, or that I've made some decisions on unresolved topics. Or maybe, I've just completely changed the plans for an upcoming meeting!

When I run, it seems that great ideas and answers just surface to my brain. It's as if all the pros and cons that have been weighing on me get sorted out in the cadence of my steps. As a result, when I know that I have to make a big decision, it's off to the park or the trails to figure it all out.

One such time was when I was thinking about winding down a long magazine publishing career. There was an upcoming management change, and although I would benefit from a promotion, I thought it might be time to do something new.

As I ran the streets of New York, it gave me the clarity to sort out the pros and cons of the decision. Fortunately, my father and his only brother, my uncle, were both in New York at the time—my uncle on a visit from Australia, my dad from Pennsylvania. This gave me the chance to talk to two people who I knew always had my best interest in mind.

It's as if all the pros and cons that have been weighing on me get sorted out in the cadence of my steps.

"You've had a great publishing career," my dad said. "Are you really ready to leave?"

"Give the new management some time," my uncle added, sharing how he had had a similar moment in his career many years before. I took in all of the input and went out for a run to sort it out.

My new boss, David, was someone who I had known in the industry. He was an accomplished publishing executive who I had always admired. We had even worked together for a short time in another company.

Finishing up a six-mile loop in Central Park, the decision was made. I'd give it a shot for a year to see how it would all transpire. Ultimately, I realized that I still loved my industry, the company that I worked for, and the incredibly talented team of leaders that I had assembled, a group that I truly believed was the best in the business. We all had a lot more work to do and new heights to achieve. It took me less than 6 weeks to realize that I had made the right decision.

From the beginning, David and I clicked, he treated me as his partner and relied on my input and advice. With a lot to manage, we figured out how we would each spend our time, playing to each other's strengths and interests. We went on to spend the next 8 years together, along with others on the core team. We made many decisions, always the right choice for the business (aided by many long runs) and navigated the ups and downs of a changing media landscape. We outperformed our industry peers and established our company as the place to do good business. David and I were named the media executives of the year by one of our leading trade magazines and shared that spotlight with many of our colleagues.

That experience had allowed me to build on my knowledge and experience in so many ways, leading to a seat on my company's board of directors, thanks to our Vice Chairman and former CEO, Frank, one of my great mentors.

We all had a lot more work to do and new heights to achieve. It took me less than 6 weeks to realize that I had made the right decision.

When David announced that he was leaving his media career, it was time for another run to think about what I might do next. I didn't raise my hand to our CEO, Steve, to be considered for the job. I had spent 40 years in the magazine industry, 21 years at my company, and while I wanted to help out in the next transition, I was already running the trails to think about my own next step. It had been an amazing career for me, a working-class kid who arrived in New York with only $60 in his pocket and a dream to make a contribution. My career had fulfilled me beyond my wildest expectations.

If we are lucky in our careers, we get to work with exceptional people and inspiring leaders along the way. In my early career years, Jack was my mentor, helping me find my first publishing job at *GQ*. Later in our careers, we worked together as executive vice presidents of our company, and I followed him as the chairman of the Magazine Publishers of America, our industry trade group. Cathie, a world class leader, was my mid-career mentor. Her vision transformed our company, and I was honored to be a part of her executive team. Both of them remain close friends and advisers to this day.

From business trips to Dallas and Milan to vacation time in Santa Fe and New Zealand, running has always helped me clarify my thoughts about the future. I pondered several questions on my mind: What really mattered to me? What were my passions? What was I good at? What wasn't I good at? How often do we go into a deep soul search on these important questions, especially as we calculate how many years we have left on planet Earth?

If we are lucky in our careers, we get to work with exceptional people and inspiring leaders along the way.

After many long runs to determine what I wanted to do with the rest of my life, it all came together. I had always had a lot of interests, and I decided to put them on overdrive. Some friends and I had started a foundation, Circle of Generosity, which led to a decision to pursue a second master's degree in non-profit management at Columbia University to learn more about the philanthropy world.

Globetrotting has always been my passion, having traveled to over 120 countries and yet still having at least 20 more places on my destination list, including Papua New Guinea and Rwanda. I still had Tokyo, Chicago, and Boston to run to finish the Six Majors, not to mention other marathon destinations. Writing and photography are part of the plan. This is my 10th book with more ideas in the works.

When I talked to our CEO, Steve, about my own timing, he suggested that I stay on with the company in the role of special media adviser to him. It was a great opportunity to continue an association with a company that I loved and with a leader who had made his own mark on moving our company forward.

I had developed my plan, but one never knows how it will work out until you are in it. It's like a marathon. You know you have to cover 26.2 miles, but a lot can trip you up along the way. The key is to maintain focus, both mentally and physically, to get to the goal.

When my 86-year-old father told me that he was still searching for answers, it was an inspiration to me. You can never stop learning, and you can never stop growing. Keep thinking. Keep searching. Keep running. We all find the right answers in due time, the answers that are right for us. Ultimately, that is all that really matters.

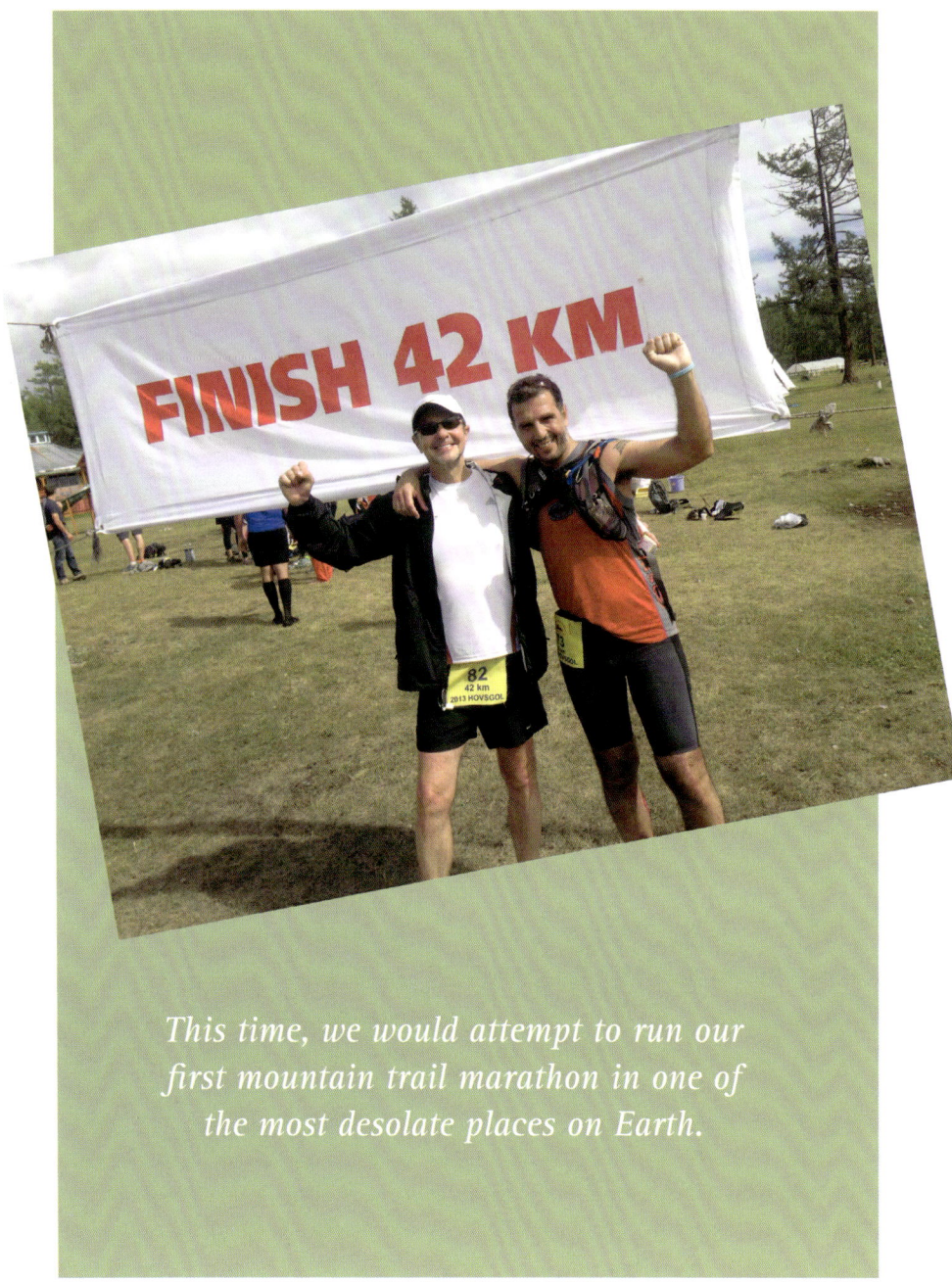

This time, we would attempt to run our first mountain trail marathon in one of the most desolate places on Earth.

Mongolia Madness

"Take your normal marathon time and add 50 percent to it. If you are lucky, that is how you will finish," said one of the organizers of the Mongolia Sunrise to Sunset Marathon held each year in Khovsgol National Park in the far north of the country.

"In the past, we had a runner break his leg, while another one fell down the mountain and broke a vertebrae," he continued, adding that a volunteer doctor would have to sign off on a medical okay in order for each of us to run. I have had many running partners over the years, but this was the first time that Fear had become my new companion.

My sister Peg and I had decided we didn't want the typical city run in the streets of Tokyo or Singapore to complete our Asia marathon. Instead, we wanted to push the envelope with a new experience. This time, we would attempt to run our first mountain trail marathon in one of the most desolate places on Earth.

We flew to Ulaanbaatar from Beijing, where we met our fellow runners from around the world, sixty-five of us total, thirty-two who would run the 42k and thirty-three who would do an ultra-marathon. From there, we took a two-hour flight to Murun, followed by a dusty van ride through the stunning mountain scenery, passing nomad villages along the way.

We arrived at Toilogt camp, situated along the lake, just as the late afternoon sun reflected on the still water as well as on the collection of yurts and teepees that would be our home for the next week. Race day was day four of our stay and until then, we would spend the days hiking and horseback riding into the forests and wide-open fields as we acclimatized for the race that, at times, would exceed seven thousand feet in altitude.

Peg and I settled into our teepee, complete with two single beds separated by a wood stove that would provide heat during the cold August nights. We learned there would be no phone service, internet, or television during our stay. We would have to resort to good, old-fashioned conversation, reading books, playing cards or board games—a throwback to what life used to be like. The camp had a communal dining room, as well as communal showers and toilets, and a small general store where we could buy basic provisions, including extra gloves and caps for the unexpected chilly air.

On the first night, as we all gathered for dinner, we did what runners always do best: we talked about our races, our stats, and our injuries, as well as how we ended up in Mongolia. Simon, a Canadian adventurer who produced and starred in a television series called *Boundless*, was part of the group. There was a father and son from Switzerland; several Americans who were living in Asia, such as Dave and California-born Joe, an American serial runner; and an assembly of other expats, like Francesco, an Italian living in China. During dinner on the first night in camp, four Italian runners in their twenties arrived full of swagger on motorcycles from Ulaanbaatar.

This time, we would attempt to run our first mountain trail marathon in one of the most desolate places on Earth.

Most everyone said they wanted an adventure, something that broke up the routine and the sometime monotony of a typical marathon. I also got the sense there was a bit of trepidation among many of the runners as they took on this unique challenge. My new friend Fear was beside me as I listened to several people talk about their runs across the Sahara or in the Andes mountains of Peru. My anxiety level rose as I realized that many of my fellow runners were leagues ahead of me with regards to experience and ability. Why did I think this was such a good idea? They had taken running to a whole different level, not necessarily focused on time but in performance within challenging circumstances.

Peg was dealing with a separate anxiety, as she was nursing a foot injury and wondering if she would be able to run at all. On our second day in the camp, the organizers suggested we hike in the area that would be the first couple of miles of the race, a narrow trail through a dense forest that had fallen trees and brush. Since we would be starting the race before dawn with headlamps for light to get us through the wooded area, they convinced us it was a practical exercise to prepare us for the beginning of the course.

We also learned that we would carry backpacks, complete with whistles and notepads to write down our numbers should we get injured and be discovered by a local in the mountains. The pack would also include an ace bandage, a Mylar blanket, a first-aid kit, some emergency food, a 1.5-liter bottle and water purifiers should we need to get water from the lake or other sources, and raingear since it could rain or snow in the mountains.

On the run, there would be no chips, no time or mileage markers, and no spectators. We would be out in the wilderness, following green paint markers on trees and rocks as our navigational guide. There would be three aid stations on the route, one at 12.5k, one at 25k, and the last at 32k. At each station, race volunteers would mark down our number to keep track of us, give us some food and water, and check our overall well-being. We were told they had the right to pull us out of the run if they felt that exhaustion or delirium had set in.

My confidence was so sufficiently eroded that I wondered if I would ever be able to complete such a challenging course. All of a sudden, running Tokyo, a normal city marathon on flat roads, seemed like it would have been a much smarter choice! Maybe I hadn't done enough research or focused on the details, but there I was in the middle of nowhere with nothing else to preoccupy my time except get my head around how I would find the courage and stamina to conquer this newfound feeling of fear that permeated my whole being.

What I had learned about other fearful situations in the past was that I had to figure out how to confront the fear head-on. And I needed to do it fast, as the race was two days away. As Mark Twain said, "Courage is resistance to fear, mastery of fear, not absence of fear!" What is true is that misery loves company, or put another way, company can help make fear less miserable if you build a community of supporters to get through it.

> *What I had learned about other fearful situations in the past was that I had to figure out how to confront the fear head-on.*

It became apparent that everyone was feeling a bit anxious, evident when the gallows humor set in. Who would fall down the mountain? When we learned there could be wolves on the course, we identified who would be the most delicious runner to eat. Since there wasn't a lot of body fat in this group, we laughed that maybe the wolves would be discouraged and leave. We began to form our own small community, talking through our fears and committing to help each other to be safe through the treacherous terrain.

When the organizers suggested we find a running buddy, allowing us to run the whole race together, I matched up with Francesco, the Italian living in Guangzhou, China. Peg joined up with Ashlyn, an Irish woman living in Shanghai, who ironically was born and raised twenty minutes from the village in County Monaghan where our grandfather was born a century ago. A group of us—a New Zealander, an American from

Michigan, and Joe, who was wrapping up a business experience in China—bonded over a standing card game each afternoon. We speculated about the dangers of the course, wondering what it would really be like up in the mountains, especially since we still had no real clue what to expect.

One of the reasons I decided on this race was that I wanted to become more of myself, which was to be a true adventurer. When I hit forty, I had decided to start pursuing different adventures to push my own limits and test my abilities. When someone asked me to define myself, one of the adjectives that I wanted to include would be *adventure traveler*. Twenty years later, I had ventured to the jungles of Madagascar, the Himalayas, Patagonia, and to Antarctica and the Arctic in pursuit of experiences. Running a marathon in Mongolia seemed to fit the bill for this self-identification. But none of my past exploits had ever instilled actual fear in me. This would be Adventure 2.0!

On race day, we had a wakeup call at 2:30 a.m., followed by an assembly in the dining room for some tea and breakfast of eggs and toast. Each of us had to make sure we had all our supplies in order, as well as make sure we had the proper clothing. Some of the runners wore shoes that were a hybrid of running shoes and mountain hikers, but I was committed to my regular running shoes, along with a pair of breathable socks, shorts, a long sleeve shirt under raingear, and a singlet rolled up in my backpack.

As we gathered for the race under a makeshift starting line banner, we were joined by ten Mongolians who would run, too. As locals who train in the mountains, I suspected we'd never see them again once the race started, as they were used to these conditions. Under the clear, moonlit sky, I realized Fear was next to me. My plan was to somehow tame him, losing him along the way, as I would a running jacket that might become too burdensome to carry.

But none of my past exploits had ever instilled actual fear in me. This would be Adventure 2.0!

As the countdown for the race began, I took a deep breath and then bang—we were off. Francesco, Ashlyn, Peg, and I decided to start together, along with Joe and Dave. We headed into the woods, a trail of bouncing headlamps illuminating the dense forest. A few runners tripped and fell over fallen trees. I decided to yell, "Tree down!" anytime I jumped over one. Since Peg had decided the day before to ignore her foot injury and attempt the race anyway, I was particularly concerned about her. While we don't typically run at the same pace, we stayed together at the start of the race as the noise of branches cracking and runners' grunts broke the stillness of the predawn air.

With each step, I looked down to avoid tripping or falling, something that had never been on my mind in the streets of Philadelphia or Buenos Aires. There were rocks and twigs and dips in the ground that kept me focused each step of the way, making sure that my shoelaces were tight and that my backpack was secure. I wasn't sure if this was going to make me a more adventurous runner, but it seemed like the beginning of a new experience.

Fear was keeping pace with me, too, and if the first mile of this course was any indication of its challenge, he was going to be with me for a long time! Suddenly, we moved out of the forest and onto a flat field cleared of any foliage. In front of us was shimmering Lake Khovsgol with just a hint of dawn breaking through the clouds above it. I took a deep breath and began to find my pace, as the group began to thin out. If I focused on steady breathing maybe that would help me manage Fear and keep it in check, I thought.

> *I wasn't sure if this was going to make me a more adventurous runner, but it seemed like the beginning of a new experience.*

Francesco and I gave each other a supportive nod, and I looked over at Peg, who gave me a thumbs-up, a good sign that her foot wasn't bothering her. My sister, a personal trainer, is tough and always plows through any situation to conquer it, so I was confident she would somehow find her way to the finish.

"Don't forget to look out for wolves," Joe yelled as he quickened his pace.

"Keep your backpack snug," someone else shouted.

Like any regular marathon, the goal in the beginning is to find the pace that is right for you. "Run your own race," my longtime running friend Keith had always advised me.

Knowing I was going to face some mountainous terrain, I decided on an easy pace going out, an 11-minute mile, to conserve energy. Since this was not a race for time, another strange concept to me, it seemed like the smart thing to do. I did a quick inventory of my body to make sure there were no quirky pains or aches, the kinds of problems that can sometimes appear out of nowhere during a race.

In my head, I visualized I was out for an early morning run in Central Park as a way to get my mind off of what was actually in my future on this journey. But at the same time, I wanted to be present for the actual race, to appreciate where I was in the world. My mind was on reaching the 10k mark, generally the moment when I have committed to a pace, usually around a 9-minute mile. At that time, I can start focusing on what I always hope will be a marathon finish line that is somewhere under four hours. Although, I knew that wasn't likely with this race.

My breathing was steady, and even though I was beginning to feel a little calmer, Fear was still wrapped around me. I had been secretly dreading being out on this course, and the continued anxiety of what was ahead was still there . . . and Fear knew it. In the past, I had learned the lesson that anticipation is often more full of fear than the act itself, especially when you are pushing to test yourself, and I tried to remind myself of that.

I channeled the memory of the time I did my first solo flight as a student pilot, my instructor's seat empty next to me. Once I lifted off the runway, I had an ironic sense of calm as I realized I was on my way to fulfilling my boyhood dream to be a pilot. Conscious, steady breathing helped me then, as I climbed into the open sky. In order to become who we want to be, there is sometimes fear involved. Harnessing that emotion and dissolving it in my mind had been how I broke through in the past to achieve those dreams. My formula had been to always be in the present, almost a Zen-like approach to the actual experience, taking long, deep breaths. However, that focus wasn't working for me this time.

Conscious, steady breathing helped me then, as I climbed into the open sky. In order to become who we want to be, there is sometimes fear involved.

As I arrived at the 12.5k aid station, the sun had begun to rise. Stopping for some water, I noticed two simple tables with plates of apples, tomatoes, donuts, and boiled potatoes. Next to it was an open fire with boiling water for hot tea and chicken soup. This was definitely not your typical race stop with water and Gatorade! I sipped some water and decided to grab a couple of potatoes to see how they might help. Sure enough, they gave me the boost that has now become my secret energy source for every race I've run since. Forget energy gels and protein bars. Now, I grab a few potatoes wrapped in aluminum foil and stuff them in my pockets and I nibble on them throughout a race.

As we continued on the course alongside the lake, I decided this was going to be the place to shed my ongoing fear. Another way that I had dealt with Fear in the past was to pretend I was literally removing the invisible cloak of it and finding a place to toss it away, whether it was on a mountain, an open field, or out of the window of a Cessna 172 airplane. It was how I dealt with getting rid of real, in-the-moment fear. It's not an easy solution, and for it to work, you have to allow your fear to come to the surface of your mind. Until you admit that you're scared of failing at a new endeavor and embrace it, you cannot tackle it to the ground or push it off a mountaintop. I continued to appreciate that Fear was still with me as I struggled to find how I would master it this time around.

We had been running on a dirt trail that soon turned to the left, and suddenly there it was, Chichee Pass, a mountain that rose from 5,400 feet to 7,500 feet. As we started to ascend the mountain, we realized that our slow, steady pace would become even slower. We were at a 50-degree angle, and it soon became apparent that we had to walk. Francesco and I started to race walk, catching up to Meg, a Japanese runner, and her running buddy, Linda, who was an Australian.

We were above the clouds then, and a light rain began to fall as mist moved around us. We began panting and struggling, so we decided to stay together as a small group, the wind whipping, pushing us backward, as we looked at the deep ravine below. The top of the mountain still seemed a long way off though we saw the small outlines of the front runners ahead of us. We all took one step, one breath, one step, one breath, trudging to the top, feeling our hamstrings tighten up, but we moved forward nonetheless.

The forty-five-minute walk-jog approach frustrated me, but then again, aside from some training runs in the mountains above Santa Fe, I had never attempted this altitude or incline before, so why would I think I could come out and master this course? In the past, I had always been good at assimilating new experiences once I was in them. I had stood at the top of Mount Kilimanjaro at dawn, after starting the final ascent at midnight. Skydiving and a stint of racecar driving had also taught me the importance of being in the present to achieve another level in my pursuit of being an adventurer. My Zen approach to being in the moment still hadn't kicked in for this race, however.

The thing about reaching the top of a mountain is that you then have to go down the mountain. The trail to the top had been steep, but clear of any debris. But as we looked down the other side, we realized that there was no real trail. We would have to run or walk or jog amid brush and rocks and twigs, continuing to look for the green markers that would guide us to the finish line. Meg, Linda, Francesco, and I began to descend at a light jog, cautiously watching where our feet landed. We stopped for a minute to breathe in the fresh Mongolian air and take in the stunning vista before us. The sky was now clear and sunny, and it was around fifty-five degrees. We took off our raingear and stuffed it into our backpacks and began again.

Twenty minutes into the descent, it was no longer our hamstrings that felt a burn, but rather our quadriceps. On a weeklong hiking trip to Bhutan, I had learned that going downhill was often times more challenging than going uphill. Very few marathons in the world have the kind of terrain that this one had, and yet for some reason, this marathon doesn't even make it on many of the lists of the world's most challenging runs. I made a mental note to let whomever makes these lists know that the Mongolian Sunrise to Sunset should be included. To run in the wilderness with only markings on trees and rocks made this one of the most isolated, difficult courses anywhere.

At the bottom of the mountain, we all decided to have a short rest. We re-tied our shoes, and I ate a boiled potato and drank some water. Meg and Linda decided to move on and we wished them luck with the promise of a toast to our small posse back at camp.

"Don't get eaten by any wild animals," yelled Linda as she waved goodbye.

We all took one step, one breath, one step, one breath, trudging to the top, feeling our hamstrings tighten up, but we moved forward nonetheless.

As we looked around, Francesco and I realized there were no other runners in sight. I wondered how Peg was faring with her foot problem since we separated around the 5k mark. I realized that my companion Fear was still with me; I needed to invent a new skill on the spot to deal with it. We began to jog and found ourselves in an open marsh, at times a bit watery. Looking for ways to avoid stepping into any deep holes, we moved slow. At this point, we had no idea what our time was and we didn't care. Our goal was to conserve energy, avoid accidents, and to stay dry. As we moved out of the marshy area onto a flat field, we saw one of the green markers that led us to the second aid station at 25.5k. So far, the markers had been easy to identify, allaying our prerace fears that we might get lost in the wilderness.

There, we found two volunteers with the same food offerings as the first station. I sipped some hot tea and tasted a slice of apple. Two runners were stretched out on the ground, one with his quads locked up and the other just exhausted from moving too fast on the course. Francesco and I did a buddy check. We both felt pretty good. Fear was still there with me, too, and I mumbled to myself that I would be dealing with him shortly.

We had survived Chichee only to hear from the volunteers that the second mountain was shorter but more treacherous. As I looked up at it, I knew this was going to be where Fear and I would take each other on; I was determined to win.

"Well, let's conquer this baby," I said as we began to run at a slow pace.

The run to the top of Khirvesteg Pass was 5.5k and it was steep. To add to the tension, we quickly came upon a trail that was about two feet wide along a cliff that overlooked a drop of several hundred feet. This was the famous spot where a runner had tripped a few years earlier and fallen down into the valley below, breaking his vertebrae. This part of the course had always been in the back of my mind.

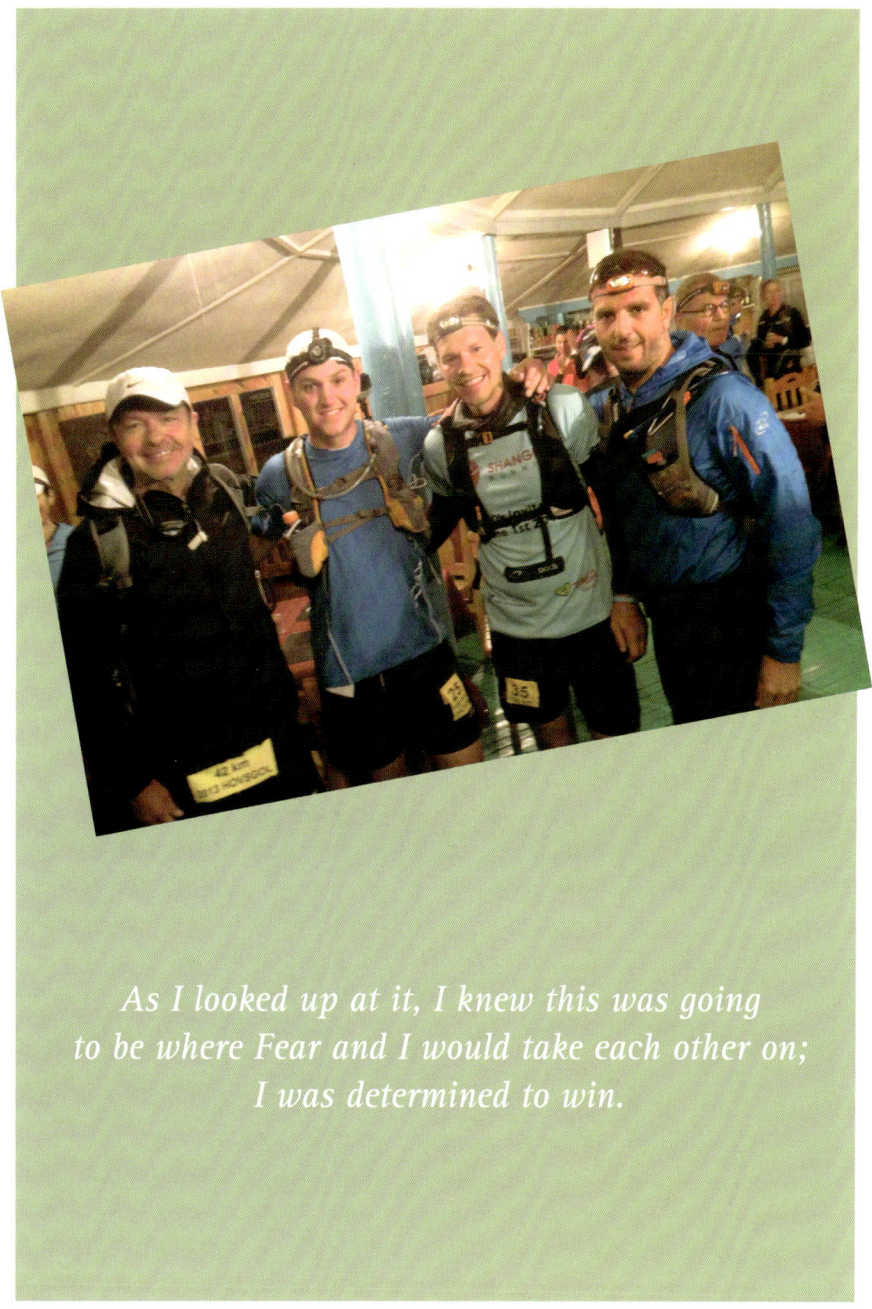

*As I looked up at it, I knew this was going
to be where Fear and I would take each other on;
I was determined to win.*

"Let's slow down a bit more," I suggested as we decided to walk/jog along the 2k stretch, wondering if there were wolves waiting below. It was here that I decided to take on Fear with a new tactic since I was feeling more confident as the race progressed. I started a conversation with him. Why was he still hanging around me? I was actually doing pretty well so far, so why was I even letting him stick around? There didn't seem to be any real reason to have him there. I had actually been losing my fear along the way but hadn't completely realized it. I looked around at the gorgeous Mongolian scenery, put myself back into the present of being there, took a deep breath, and told Fear that he would have to leave now!

Then we were off the cliff trail, taking a left turn to head up what was an even steeper hill than we had thought. Fear decided to hang around just a little bit longer! After a few minutes running up the hill, we found ourselves on all fours, literally crawling up the mountainside.

To add to the tension, we quickly came upon a trail that was about two feet wide along a cliff that overlooked a drop of several hundred feet.

"This isn't a marathon," said Francesco, "this is crazy stuff."

All I could do was give him a nervous laugh in response. We passed another runner sitting on a rock on the hillside, exhausted. He waved us on, saying that he needed to rest, and I took some quiet satisfaction in noting that it was one of the Italian twenty-somethings who had been a bit cocky back in the camp. The forty-five-minute climb/crawl/hike to the top of that mountain was one of the most strenuous things I have ever done in my life. With my legs wobbling and my head pounding, my internal chant became, "You can do this!" It was also the place that I wrestled Fear off my back as I plowed through the challenge of scaling that mountain.

As we tumbled to the top, we stood there breathing hard, raising our arms above our heads to stretch, to yell out our exhaustion in a primal scream. During the ascent, Francesco was actually doing better than me, and I had urged him to go on.

"No way," he said, "We are doing this together to the very end." That was the moment I knew we would get through this as a pair, even if it meant crawling our way to the end. There is nothing like a committed friend to help you through those difficult stretches in life.

At the top of the mountain was a Mongolian Ovoo, a shrine built by the locals to honor the spirits of the land. Back at the camp, we were told by the organizers to circle it either once or three times clockwise for good luck. Both of us decided that three times seemed appropriate, and we let out some whoops as we danced around the circle. It was during that ritual that I took the invisible cloak of fear and decided it was time to finally and completely peel if off and throw it off the mountaintop.

"Good-bye, Fear," I yelled, ending the dialog I had started with him a few kilometers earlier.

As we gazed out at the stunning scenery, we realized the most daunting part of the race was behind us. It was that feeling when you know you're on the other side of a challenge. And now that Fear was gone, I felt lighter and confident. It's funny that even though you know how amazing you'll feel when you get rid of fear, that alone isn't enough to help you get rid of it in the first place.

As we jogged down the hillside, watching for rocks and brush, we looked for the 32k aid station, which would be our marker that we were only 10k from the finish line. Arriving at the station, we learned that this stop was only a lone man with a barrel of water to refill our bottles. I popped a potato in my mouth, took a few swigs of water, and asked Francesco how he was feeling. All he could say is that he was glad the worst was behind us, and I agreed. We decided to keep our pace easy and enjoy the rest of the race along the flat dirt trail. At times, this was tough due to our exhaustion, but we pushed each other along, stopping occasionally to stretch a bit.

Off in the distance, we saw Lake Khovsgol and the finish line. It was a beautiful day, crystal clear skies and pure air. I wondered how Peg was doing and also wondered how the ultra-marathoners could possibly run a second marathon. We crossed the finish line together, our hands clasped in friendship; we lifted them into the air as a volunteer yelled, "That was six hours and forty-seven minutes!" A dozen or so people, including Meg and Linda, had assembled at the finish line to cheer us on, and Francesco and I patted each other on the back in a congratulatory embrace.

After some hot soup and tea, we joined the group at the finish line, cheering each runner as they came in. Peg completed the course just before nine hours, her injury still there but with her own fear conquered. When she got home, she learned she had a slight hairline fracture, which had probably been there since before the race. For the other marathoners, one got lost, and although found, never finished the race. For the 100k runners, four had to drop out, but we celebrated them, too. That night, there was a ceremony of medals given to recognize our accomplishment and we ate and drank into the wee hours of the morning.

We had become a band of runners, bonded forever. We've stayed in touch via Facebook, cheering Dave on during his marathon in North Korea and reaching his goal of running on all seven continents. Francesco and I email each other regularly, and when Joe came back to the United States, we struck up a lasting friendship. We reminisced about our great adventure together over drinks and dinner at a Manhattan restaurant.

I couldn't even conjure up the fear that had been with me when I first arrived at the camp four days earlier. Running a mountain marathon had taught me to confront Fear in a new way. What I realized is that his appearance on the scene had been permitted by me. I let him in only because I was about to experience something I had never done before. My own self-doubt about taking on this new kind of running adventure opened the door to my relationship with him. In hindsight, all I needed to do was reinforce my own love of running as the core of what I was about to do; it was just different terrain. The fundamentals were all the same, but I had let myself be hijacked by the anxiety of the unknown.

Fear is a metaphor for so many challenges that we face in life, and it was a reminder to always get back to the core of who you are and what you love to do. I now feel confident about running the Sahara or the Andes and have set my sights on the Everest Base Camp Marathon, which is a two-week hike up the mountain, and then a 42k run down. Fear may want to come along on that trip, too, but now I have the courage to resist him.

Whenever I find myself fearful about something in life, I close my eyes and take myself back to the mountains of Mongolia. I picture myself crawling up that mountainside, or moving along the cliff trail, and I remember how I shoved Fear out. He will never truly go away, but when he comes to visit, I know how to manage him. My next goal is to uninvite him from the very beginning of the experience. When I master that, I know a whole new set of adventures will be possible.

Mark Twain knew what he was talking about when it comes to Fear. It only takes courage to master it and to resist it. And when you do, you are free to be who you are and become who you want to be. This marathon had taught me that lesson.

Move Over, Penguins,
Marathon Coming Through

At the tail end of the most bone-chilling winter in recent years, I left New York for Antarctica, the coldest and driest place on Earth, where the sun never completely sets.

It is—and feels—truly at the end of the world. The terrain, so to speak, is 98 percent thick, continental ice sheet and 2 percent barren rock, an otherworldly landscape of glaciers and penguin rookeries accessible via inflatable boat that you must take from your ship, which doubles as your hotel.

A trip there promises an extreme adventure that is like bait to hardy travelers, but it's safe to say that the eighty-six of us who went on a tour there this March were among the hardiest who visit: we were there to run a marathon. The race would be the culmination of my quest to run seven marathons in seven years on seven continents.

That may sound ambitious, but it was not a long-held dream of mine. I stumbled upon this challenge when my younger sister, Peg, called me seven years ago to ask if I would run a marathon with her. It would be her first.

I was a veteran, having finished four, but was out of practice because I hadn't run one in more than thirty years; my last had been New York City. "I just might have another one in me," I said, wondering how I would do now that I was in my fifties. It would be to embrace, in the words of Teddy Roosevelt, "the strenuous life."

In the years between the marathons of my mid-twenties and the one I had run with Peg, I had fully embraced adventure travel. I climbed Mount Kilimanjaro, went on Himalayan treks in Nepal and Bhutan, hiked glaciers in Patagonia, and more. But adding a marathon to off-the-beaten-path places seemed like adventure travel 2.0, compounding both the challenge and the reward. Run Safaricom, a race through an African game park amid wild animals? Why not?

In my post-marathon years, I continued to run, but usually not more than ten miles, so it took me a good six months to get up to speed for the first one.

Peg and I chose London as our inaugural marathon in 2008, followed by Buenos Aires, the Gold Coast of Australia, and Philadelphia. Then we kicked it up a bit with

Kilimanjaro, in Tanzania, and then our first trail marathon in northern Mongolia, the most challenging course we had ever run.

When I learned that, because of growing demand, there was a three-year waiting list for Antarctica, I signed up in order to make it the last of the seven continents. In doing so, I would join the elite club of 410 others who had taken the same challenge, according to Thom Gilligan, who owns Boston-based Marathon Tours, the group that organizes the Antarctica run. But first I had to complete the race. The other marathoners and I met up in Buenos Aires in March and flew to Ushuaia, at the bottom tip of Argentina, to board the *Akademik Ioffe*, a Russian vessel built for scientific research that would be our home for ten days.

The first two days on the ship were spent crossing the Drake Passage, which can be treacherous. While most of us were wearing a transdermal patch to prevent seasickness, the crossing affected at least twenty passengers, keeping the ship's doctor busy. The race was scheduled for the fifth day, allowing everyone to stabilize. We spent our downtime getting to know one another, listening to lectures on Antarctica, and reading. Like almost all my fellow runners, I had traveled alone, which meant I'd get a roommate. Mine was Andro, a New Zealander who was also hoping to complete his own seven on seven.

"I have always needed to have a challenge and this seemed like the perfect one," he told me.

Staging a marathon on the continent has had its challenges over the years. When Mr. Gilligan conceived the idea, he had to select a location that would not only provide a course that could be marked out and not destroyed by the weather, but also be easily accessible in case of emergency. That place was King George Island (just north of the Antarctic Peninsula), where we ran through or near four different scientific bases operated by four different countries. As a working island, it offered some roads, communication, and an evacuation route, since medivac insurance was a requirement on this trip.

Still, there have been hiccups. The first marathon took place in 1995, and one was scheduled every other year until 2001, when conditions were so bad the race took place on the ship, as runners did 422 laps to get to 26.2 miles. In 2013, the run was cancelled when the ship was damaged by an iceberg, then rescheduled a few weeks later. Even so, the course had become so icy that a number of runners slipped and broke collarbones, cracked ribs, and faced minor hypothermia.

Our course involved six legs. We would run 2.18 miles toward the Uruguayan base through hills and mud and ice, return to where we started, head west for 2.18 miles through the Russian base, then the Chilean and Chinese bases for the turnaround. That

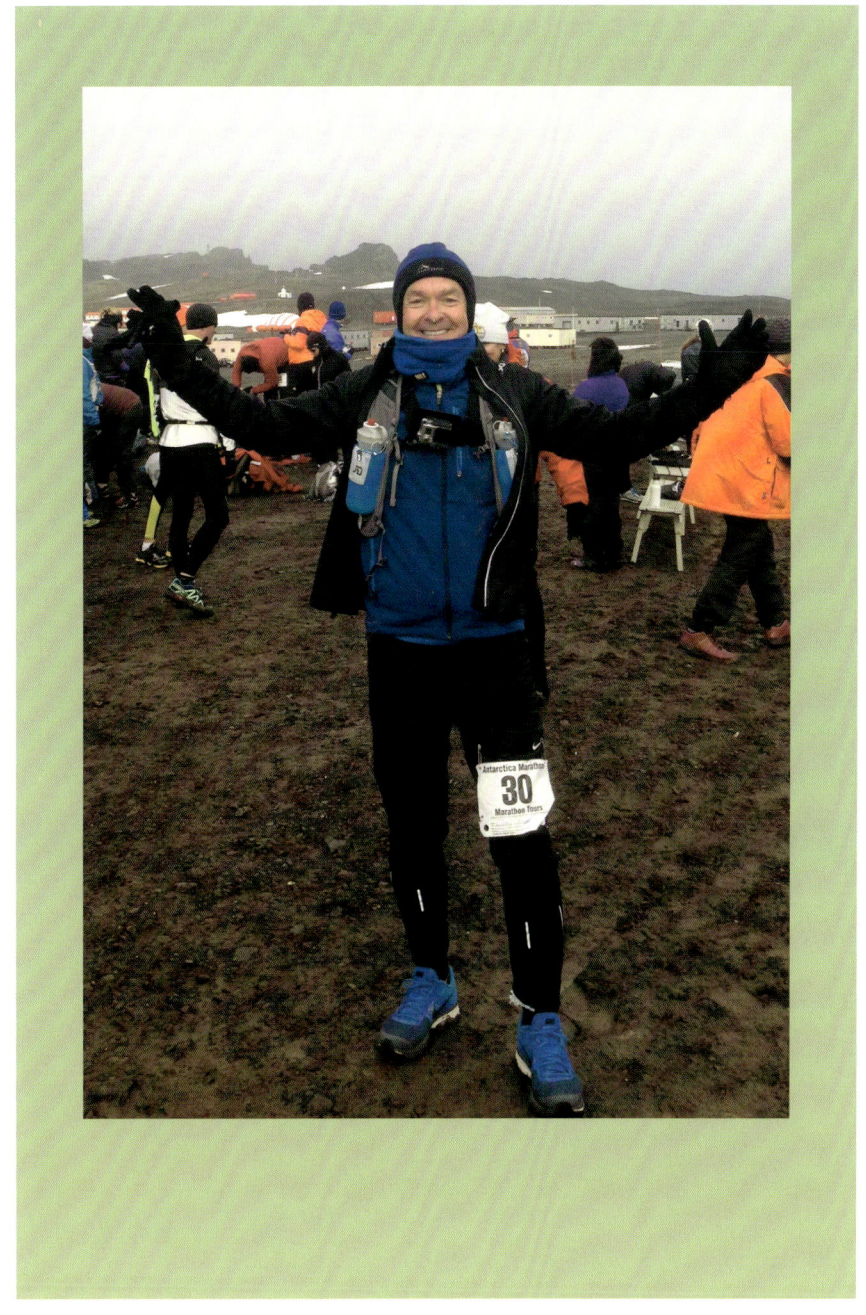

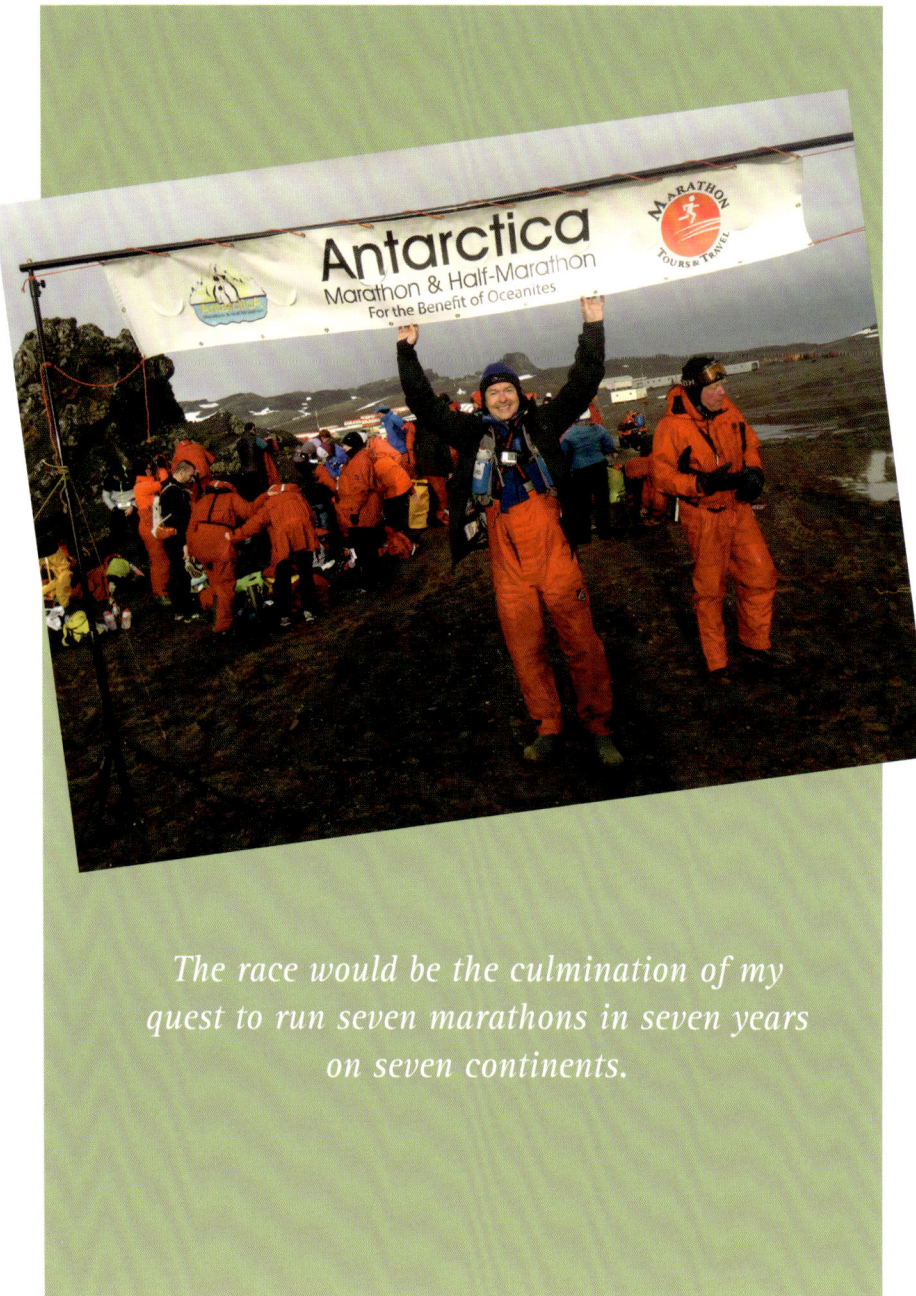

The race would be the culmination of my quest to run seven marathons in seven years on seven continents.

course had hills, and long stretches of rocky road there were exposed to fierce winds. We would do these legs six times to complete the marathon.

For safety, a team on ATVs would traverse the course to spot anyone in trouble.

Jenny Hadfield, a running coach and part of the crew, was there to give us some guidance. "Do not think about pace," she said. "Time means nothing on this course. It's all about energy management. Tune in to the terrain. Be mindful of the weather. Think ice, snow, mud."

It began to sink in that although we might be well trained and injury-free, there was no guarantee that we would finish.

Race day started with a 6:15 wakeup call as we assembled in the ship's mudroom, layering on rain gear over our running clothes and rubber boots until we reached the starting line.

> *It began to sink in that although we might be well trained and injury-free, there was no guarantee that we would finish.*

At 7:30, we headed down the gangplank into the inflatables. The temperature was thirty degrees, but it started to rain, the first of what would be more than a dozen climate changes we would face during the run, including a wind-chill factor that created subfreezing conditions. Stepping out of the boat into icy water, we hiked up a hill to the starting point, where we faced patches of deep mud. We searched for dry land so we could strip off our rain gear and boots to rearrange our actual race clothes and shoes.

"Make sure you double-tie your shoes," Mr. Gilligan said. "It is possible to have them sucked right off of your feet if you step into a deep mud hole."

The race began up a long hill coated with ice and snow, and within the first mile, most of us were walking up the slick, steep incline. As we moved into the course, it became apparent that there would be a lot of ice, mud, puddles, and streams (I stopped counting streams and puddles after twenty-five).

The way the course was laid out, we all passed one another multiple times, making up for the fact that there were no spectators. We supported one another on what would at times be lonely and desolate stretches on the course. For this race, a runner could decide to stop at a half marathon and earn a medal, but if you decided to go on, then you had to finish within six and a half hours, or be listed as DNF (did not finish).

Five of us had started together: Andro, Marius from Poland, Annie from Miami, and Jay from North Dakota. Like many of the runners, we had left families or partners behind to pursue our goal and had become an ad hoc family, warning each other about upcoming mud holes or big rocks.

We tried to take in the stunning scenery of glaciers, icebergs, and snowcapped mountains in the distance, but most of our time was spent looking at where we would place our feet. Surviving without a twisted ankle or a bad fall quickly became our first priority.

At Mile 17, I was ready to quit. My hands were freezing, I was exhausted and hungry and many runners had already opted out. I was done with marathoning.

"Get on with it," I said to myself. I reached into my jacket for a banana, careful to put the skin back into the pocket, drank some water, and built up my resolve. The strenuous life. I kept going.

On the fifth leg, the winds were at forty miles per hour, and I still had to run out to the far reaches of the China base. On the way back, at Mile 24, it hit me. Not the classic runner's wall, but something worse. It was a mental and physical disequilibrium that seemed to overtake me.

I had known this was going to be different than a run on the streets of New York, but nothing had prepared me for what I was experiencing. *I will not run another one of these*, I promised myself.

As I crossed the finish line, that feeling, which I can only describe as simply brutal, was joined by another: elation.

Sixty-five marathoners completed the course that day, including the five of us who started together and one who fell unconscious when he crossed the finish line. Nineteen opted for the half marathon, and one dropped out. The lead runner, Alex from Switzerland, came in at 3:56, nearly ninety minutes longer than his usual marathon time because of what we learned was one of the muddiest and wettest courses ever. My time was 5:46, placing me in the first half of the finishers. Twelve of us earned our stripes of seven marathons on seven continents.

As we headed home through the Drake, I found myself already considering the next one. I felt ready for anything. Maybe the Sahara? The Inca Trail? My mind and body had been stretched beyond what I thought was my capacity. I'd finished seven on seven, but I wasn't done. *The strenuous life* was my new mantra.

Michael Clinton © 2014 *The New York Times*

The Irish Surprise

More than forty years since there had been any contact with our Irish family, my sister Peg and I decided to search for our roots there. It had all started with our decision to run the Dublin marathon, a stop on our quest to run races around the world from Mongolia to Argentina.

Ireland was a natural choice since it was the birthplace of our paternal grandparents. Little did I know at the time that it would have a profound impact on me in ways I could have never expected.

My grandfather Louis was swept up by the excitement of the 1922 Irish Civil War, joining the Garda Síochána (Civic Guard), the police force established for the Irish Free State. He served for six years in his native county, Monaghan, before emigrating to New York City to join his older brother, Bernard, who had left Ireland in 1912.

When Louis got to New York, he learned that his brother had died, leaving him alone in a strange country with no family. The only thing we have been able to piece together about Bernard was that he had left Ireland on a ship named *Columbia* and landed in America with fifty dollars in his pocket. Beyond that, there is no information about his fifteen years in the United States since he never married, had children, or left any trace of his life here.

My grandmother, Chrissy, arrived in America in 1929. Originally from Kilkenny, she followed two sisters to New York, where she met my grandfather, thirteen years her senior, at a community Irish dance club on the Upper West Side. They married two years later, giving birth to my father, Joseph, and then his brother, Louis.

At my grandfather's funeral, my dad learned we had relatives in Monaghan with whom our family made contact, ultimately leading to a visit from me when I was twelve years old.

My cousin Vera picked me up at Shannon Airport and drove me to Monaghan, two hours north. I learned about Gaelic football, tea time, and farming the Irish countryside. She took me on trips to the west coast, exploring the Cliffs of Moher, Galway, Connemara, and Donegal, where I absorbed the beauty of the country. But there wasn't much information about either my grandfather or Bernard and why they left for America. Shortly thereafter, our family lost touch for no other reason than the preoccupation with our own lives.

Forty-five years later, I was ready to "rediscover" our family. I wanted to celebrate my immigrant roots, especially since we live in a time when there is so much debate about immigration policies. Plus, I was curious if anyone was still in Monaghan, even though my internet search came up empty.

The Dublin Marathon was one of my favorite races of all times. First of all, the Irish people are warm and friendly. The race takes place in October when the air is crisp and perfect for running. My characterization to people is that it is a midsize marathon (only twenty thousand runners!) versus the big ones like Berlin or New York. Started in 1980, the race course is mostly flat and provides every runner with a grand tour of this capital city of the Republic of Ireland, established as far back as the seventh century.

Starting at Fitzwilliam Square in the City Center, the course is a circuitous route through the center of town, with a great stretch through Phoenix Park, one of the largest enclosed parks in all of Europe. It is incredibly well organized, with water stations in ten locations, lots of markers to help celebrate the course, and a rousing crowd of spectators that will cheer you on and even try to convince you to jump into a pub to have a Guinness.

Several days before the race, we decided to take the eighty-minute drive directly to Garron, the town where my grandfather was born. My dad had told us to go to the local Catholic church, as he had heard that the priests were always a good source of information about families in the area. At St. Patrick's in the neighboring village of Tyholland, we found some tombstones with our family name, an encouraging sign we were on the right trail. As we entered the church, we met an elderly man who turned out to be the long-time caretaker.

"We're Clintons from America, looking for our family. Do you know anyone in the area?" I asked.

Pausing for a moment, he said, "Well, Seamus Clinton lives in Monaghan town and his daughters Pauline and Suzanne live up that hill," pointing to a road across from the church.

"I remember meeting a Seamus when I was a kid," I told Peg. "It must be the same person. Let's drive up to Pauline's house and knock on the door." No one was home so we left a note in the mailbox that we might be her family visiting from America.

"Well, all we can do is wait. Let's go check into the hotel, " I said.

After an early evening run around the grounds of Castle Leslie, I returned to my room to find a message from Suzanne.

"Hello, Michael. What a wonderful surprise. Will you come and visit us tomorrow morning?" she asked.

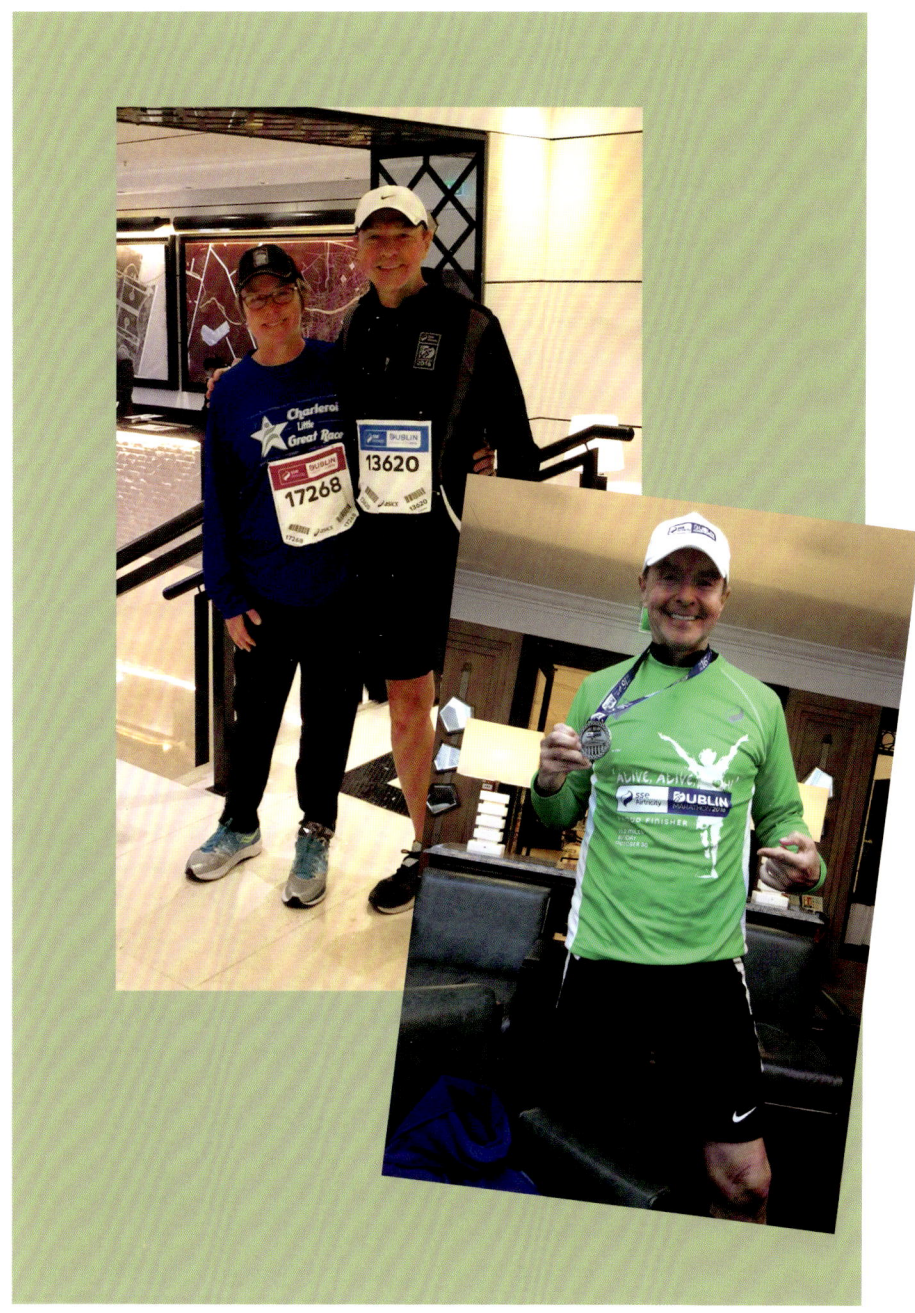

The next morning, I went out for a run by myself and wondered what we would learn about our family that day. Running around the grounds of Castle Leslie in Glaslough was the perfect place to anticipate all that we were about to experience.

Suzanne greeted us with her two-year-old son, Lugh, named after a Celtic God in Irish mythology. Pauline was there, as was her cousin Trish and father, Seamus, now a seventy-four-year-old retired councilman, whom I had met more than forty years earlier!

We all embraced and looked into each other's eyes, hardly believing what was happening. Suzanne served us tea and Irish soda bread while starting the family storytelling. After earning her degree in Natural Science in Dublin, she had been drawn back to Monaghan with her husband, Eoin, to be closer to the family and also to become its historian. She had spread out family photos, including ones of my grandfather and Bernard before they left home.

> *Little did I know at the time that it would have a profound impact on me in ways I could have never expected.*

There was a family tree dating back to the early 1800s, medals from the wars, and letters from my grandmother to her sister-in-law, telling her of the birth of my father and uncle. While holding these worn, handwritten notes from a woman I'd never met, I got a sense of what she was like, and a wave of emotion came over me.

As we went through the family history of aunts and uncles and cousins, I learned that most everyone had been farmers, but there were councilmen and property owners and nurses. But what was also revealed was something that hit me in a profound way:

In my entire life, I had never had the desire to be a father, nor had my brother, Joe. At times, there had been soul-searching moments as to why, but ultimately, I just realized it was my own sensibility.

That day in my cousin's kitchen, I learned that for generations there had been many people in our family who had no children.

My grandfather had four siblings who were childless. His brother Jim had six children, and four of them had no children. His son Seamus had six children, and two of them had no children. For the first time in my life, I was learning not only where I came from, but who I came from. It seemed to be our nature as a family that many of us just choose not to have children. That moment of truth answered a lifelong question in my own mind, as I found kindred spirits among my ancestors.

"Would you like to see the house that your grandfather was born in?" Seamus asked.

"Is it still around?" asked Peg, who was equally stunned that we had found such a treasure trove of our family's background. "Can we run there?" she asked, thinking it would be a nice warmup before the race.

"We can walk there; it's less than half a mile away! The family has owned it since the mid-1800s. Before that, we think it was an inn on the road from Monaghan town to Armagh. I raised my kids in that house," said Seamus.

How had I never known this? I wondered. I didn't remember visiting this house as a boy. Over the years, the family had acquired nearly forty acres of land around the Garron house, some of it through marriage with the Finnegans. The in-laws call the area Clintonville.

Standing in the now empty house, I asked if Vera, the cousin who had taken care of me when I visited as a boy, was still alive.

"Well, she actually turned ninety yesterday," Suzanne replied to my amazement. She had just moved into a nursing home and was having a hard time recognizing anyone, but we agreed we would go see her the next day.

Vera had been a doting aunt to her eight nieces and nephews, since she had no children of her own, and now Pauline and Trish, both of whom have no children, have picked up that family tradition for the next generation. I could relate as the uncle of eight American nieces and nephews who I indulge on a regular basis.

The next day, we went to see Vera, and while her blue eyes still sparkled, she didn't know me. As I held her hand and told her of my memories of being with her, all she did was give me a puzzling smile, and I regretted not being in touch over the years.

As we arrived in Dublin, we met our cousin Noel and Claire, his wife, embracing them as if we'd known each other our whole lives. They had lived in New Zealand, but returned home, marrying on a hill above Garron, overlooking my grandfather's house. They shared that they weren't sure if they wanted children of their own, either, but loved having a big family around them.

On a gorgeous Irish morning, we ran the Dublin marathon to the cheers of the crowd. Through the streets and parks and neighborhoods, I celebrated my newly appreciated Irishness. As I took in the neighborhoods and the beautiful people, it was as if the city embraced me and told me I belonged to them. A deep sense of belonging grew within me as I ran each mile, and I decided that I would never lose our family connection again.

Since that trip, I've returned to meet the whole family, including children of the next generation, named Aiofe and Ciara and Roan. They are proud Irish kids who are studying the Irish language and culture of their country. Some of them have a desire to visit America, but their hearts remain in Garron. Sitting around a family gathering, I felt as though I could have been with my own American family in that moment: the laughter and mannerisms were the same. Seamus could easily be my father's brother instead of his first cousin, and his son, Brian, had the same sense of humor as my brother, Joe.

Since that trip, my eighty-six-year-old father and his wife, Kathleen, have traveled to Monaghan to meet his relatives for the first time and stand in the house where his father was born. My nephew Bobby, during his time as a doctoral student in pharmacy, did a five-week course in Dublin, a choice that helped create a next-generation family connection. While there is talk about restoring the family house in Garron, I've also dreamed about owning there, a place where our family can come together to embrace their heritage and build a future together.

I've secured my Irish citizenship, a birthright thanks to my grandfather, for no other reason than to strengthen my bond there. Suzanne and I continue to search for clues about the mysterious Uncle Bernard. We will probably never know the true reason my grandfather boarded a ship in search of a new life, but like many immigrants before him, I'm sure it was the promise of what America stands for as a land of freedom and opportunity.

His decision to leave nearly one hundred years ago had led me full circle back to where it had been made. It had also given me a deeper appreciation that, as Americans, we all came from somewhere else and carry a part of that with us.

On my last trip to Garron, I went out for an early morning run through the rolling hills, past farmlands with stone fences and green pastures filled with sheep and cows. I took it all in, breathing the cool Irish mist in the air, a sense of peace settling over me, marveling at how my love of running had led me to this rich family connection. Now, I always tell people to go run a race where their forefathers came from. You never know what you might discover.

Upon returning to Suzanne's house, I discovered a big Irish breakfast waiting. Pauline had come over, along with Noel and Claire, who were staying with her. Brian and his wife, Orla, and their four kids had come to share in the conversation, along with Seamus.

We talked about my father's trip and what dreams the next generation had about their Irish futures—the kind of talk that any family would have at a Sunday morning breakfast. When it was time to leave, there were hugs and tears, and it was Brian who said, "When are you coming home again, Michael?"

In so many ways, I had come home. In fact, it seemed as if I'd always lived there.

An Interview with my (Running) Sister

My sister Peg, a personal trainer who runs her own fitness studio, decided to become a runner at forty. Since then, she has run eight marathons. Here is her story.

Q. You called me to tell me you wanted to run your first marathon. My questions at the time were: "When did you start running, and why a marathon right out of the gate?"
A. It was a week between Christmas and the New Year, and my client, Katie, had recently finished the San Francisco Marathon, and I thought, *If she can do it, I can.* I never ran in my life and had just turned forty and thought this was good a goal as any. I started running on a treadmill that day in two-minute increments. It was so very difficult, but I was determined. I knew I could do it with discipline! My intention was train for one marathon, run it, and not run again. Just a goal of one marathon. I called you that week and asked if you would run one with me, and it was game on!

Q. We decided to run the London Marathon one year out from that conversation. How did you start your running regime to get ready? What did you learn in that year of being a new runner?
A. I got books, a subscription to running magazines, spoke with other runners, and did as much web research as I could. My brain was a sponge. Being a personal trainer, I already knew the importance of advancing slowly, warming up, stretching, sprints, hill repeats, etc. and built my training plan. I went to the local running store and purchased socks, shoes, pants, and a good bra. I was ready to go!

Q. How did you stay the course during that year?
A. For the next year, I registered for 5ks, 10ks, and a half marathon. After the half marathon, Katie asked if, after 13.1 miles, could I have continued running. My response was a "hell no!" But the decision was made to run the marathon, regardless, and I was already conditioned and other than some minor aches and pains, the training was consuming but manageable. For that first marathon, I was extremely disciplined. While

teaching classes, I continued my strict training program and even got numerous clients to start running.

Q. How did it feel when you crossed the finish line at the London Marathon?
A. I ran past Buckingham Palace and when I crossed the finish line, I started crying. I couldn't believe I had done something so strenuous. A lovely British woman in front of me asked, "Are you alright, my love?" "I just ran a marathon," I replied in awe. I have never felt so strong and accomplished as I did after that first marathon.

Q. The original plan was to run one marathon and done! What happened?
A. We met a man in London who ran seven marathons on seven continents and thought that might be a fun goal. We decided to do that together. People often asked why I didn't just run my hometown marathon, and I always replied that it's the destination not the run that entices me. Many days, I did not want to run, but I knew the importance of conditioning to complete each marathon.

Q. What was your favorite marathon?
A. Tanzania was by far my favorite marathon. Running the streets with Christians and Muslims united and Mount Kilimanjaro ahead of me! Running through the vineyards and having the children run alongside me to motivate me was inspiring. I found a love of Coca-Cola in Tanzania; it's a great glycogen replenisher. You can keep your Gatorade!

Q. Your least favorite?
A. Mongolia was just questionable. I had a broken heel and wasn't sure if I could run, but the excitement of the eighty or so people lured me in. It was a brutal run! Crab-walking down steep hills, climbing over tree limbs and trunks, not sure if I was going the correct way. I had to make sure I was aware of the markings on the trees to guide me. I was in the middle of the forest and a man on a horse stopped me and started groping me. It was very frightening, as he did not speak my language and I did not speak his. I thought this was going to be the end of my life, killed in the middle of the Mongolian forest never to be found. Thankfully, I got away and was safe. After nine hours and numerous falls, I crossed the finish line, vowing that I would never run another marathon again!

Q. In your marathon training, you dealt with a lot of injuries, but you persevered!
A. In Australia, I ran with a broken metatarsal. That was my big toe. I saw someone go down about fifty yards from the finish line. I felt so bad that he could not complete the run after getting that far!

In Argentina, I ran with impingement of the deltoid. I had to run with my arm in the air. Think Statue of Liberty. Also, I forgot to pack a bra, which is pertinent for a woman running any marathon. In Argentina, they really do not have running bras, so this was quite a challenge, but I found one.

In Mongolia, I ran with a broken calcaneus. This was the hardest to run of them all. I would never recommend running with these injuries. I have learned so many tricks along the way, such as Imodium before a run, proper hydration and nutrition, body glide, bringing toilet paper, and never to try anything new on a run. No new food, drink, or clothing.

Q. You were all set to run your final continent, Antarctica, but as you were about to leave, you had to face some very personal issues, didn't you?
A. Antarctica was to be my seventh marathon on seven continents. I boarded a plane from Pittsburgh to Buenos Aires via Atlanta. I never made it past Atlanta. I had been struggling with alcohol addiction, something that is prevalent in our family. In Atlanta, it got the best of me. I missed my flight and knew I was in trouble both mentally and physically. I had to return to Pittsburgh, where I confronted my issues to get help. My husband and son and the rest of the family were 100 percent supportive as I found my path to sobriety and peace of mind. I've been sober for over two years and have never felt better and healthier.

Q. Well, sister Peg, you have always been one of the strongest and courageous women I know. You just never know—Antarctica may still be in your future someday!
A. You never know!

Q. What is your running career like now? Do you hope to run any more races in the future?
A. My running career is pretty much nonexistent due to my job as a personal trainer and spin instructor. If I do go out for a run, I try to take it slow and steady and just enjoy it. In the past, I always made it so intense. Now, it is just nice to go out and run a couple of miles and it doesn't matter how long it takes. If I slow down at work, I may run more again, but I think my marathon days are over.

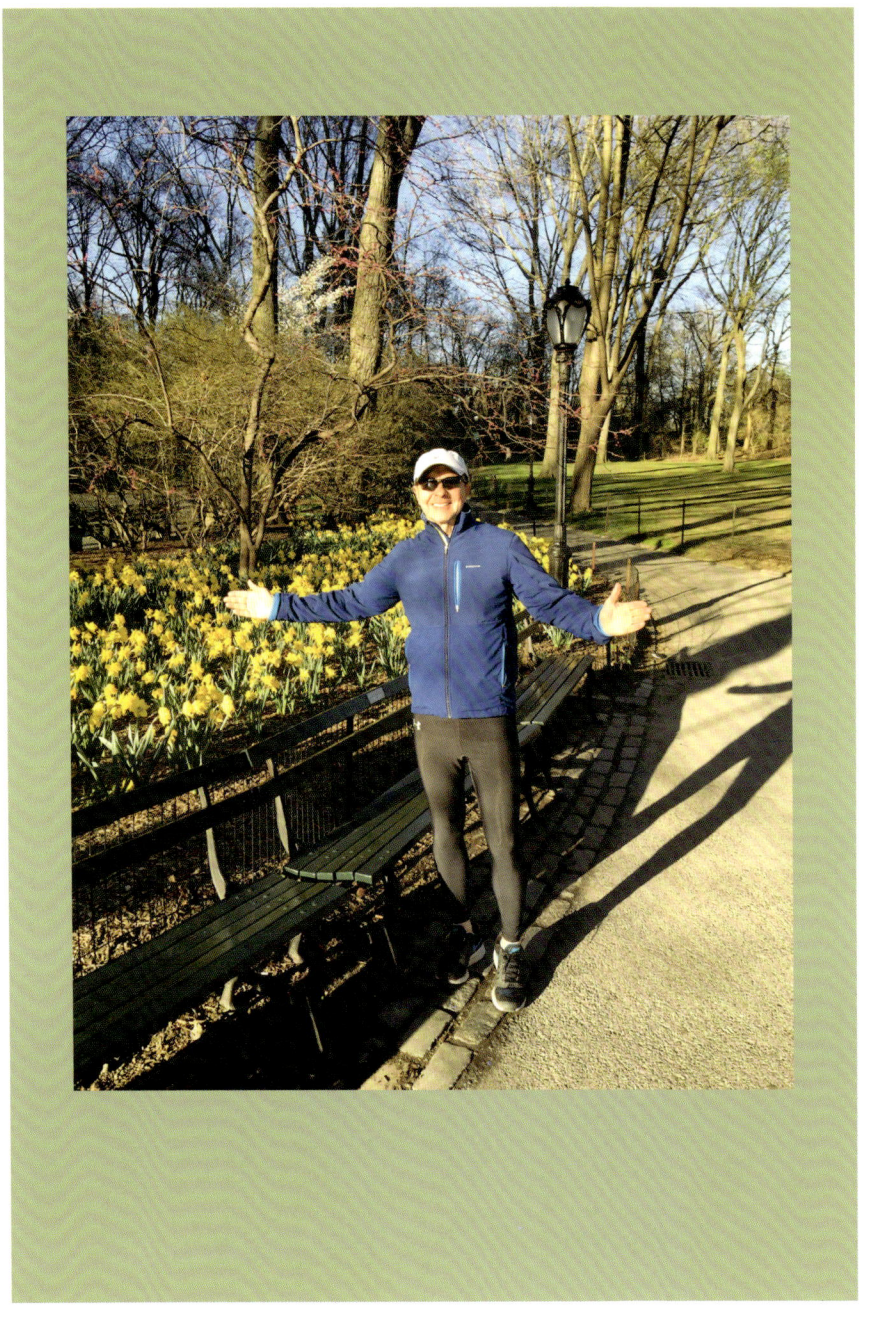

NYC: My Kind of (Running) Town

New York City is my hometown turf for running. In my mind, there's no better place to lace up and hit the streets and trails than in the city that never stops running.

Since I live three blocks from Central Park, I tell people that it's my backyard with a treasure of loops and trails and distances. For those who want an easy run, the 1.58-mile reservoir loop displays the grandeur of the city with the southern view. I've got a friend who only runs that loop three times a week for her running regimen and other friends who mix and match a course that suits their needs.

Over the years, my constant is the 6.02-mile loop within the confines of the park, but I will configure my run based on what I'm doing on any given day. Sometimes, it's a course that is five miles, sometimes it's two lower loops that add up to 3.4 miles, and on the weekends, it's exploring the hidden trails and mystery of the North Woods, where you feel like you're in the middle of a forest, miles away from the bustle of the city.

For every running visitor to New York, I tell them to head to the park for an experience that will forever endear them to my great city. Central Park is my core go-to running destination, much like New York became my core place to live, an epiphany that I had when I was ten years old. We took a family trip from our hometown in Pittsburgh to visit Manhattan, where my dad had grown up. The minute we made the descent on the highway to enter the Lincoln Tunnel, I saw the city across the Hudson River. Something clicked in my mind that it was where I belonged.

Knowing and understanding ourselves is our life's mission, and at times it can feel like a grueling run, or as my friend George advises, "Don't make the decisions of life on the uphill."

What is your core? What do you believe is right for you, and have you done the work to understand both your strengths and your weaknesses as a runner?

In the same vein, have you done the work to understand your true core? Where do you want to live? What do you want to do with your life?

Like training for a race, there are no shortcuts to go the distance with your own life. As I have always believed, go to the end of your days and work backward. What is it that you hope to achieve or leave as your legacy?

Similar to most runners, I have peaks and valleys in my running schedule. Some weeks, I realize I've only run ten miles, while other weeks, I might run thirty-five miles. Regardless of the distance, taking some type of run is always in my week's agenda.

For every running visitor to New York, I tell them to head to the park for an experience that will forever endear them to my great city.

When I'm training for a half marathon or a full marathon, it's a different story; I'm as disciplined as can be, working my runs into a morning, a lunch time, or an evening timeframe. My preference is an evening run, which allows me to burn off the stress of the day and get a second wind for the evening.

Unlike many runners, I'm not obsessed with time or running five marathons a year. I'm in awe of friends who have run fifty marathons or more, but that's not my aspiration. I know what's right for me, and a respectable one marathon a year fits my needs.

For long-distance runners, finding different routes can break up the monotony of repeating the same course over and over, and that's what makes New York City the perfect place for training. But that's also the magic of life, too. One solution may not work, so try a different one. If your life has fallen into a rut, change up your schedule to avoid stagnating. Try something new.

During my usual sixteen-week marathon training period, I keep a running diary each week as I build up to my thirteen-miler, eighteen-miler, and twenty-mile runs. I've fine-tuned my schedule to only do two eighteen-plus mile runs, when I used to do three or even four. I've bought into the new school of thought that sometimes less is more. My training schedule never exceeds forty-five miles in any given week, and it has actually improved my stamina and time during a race. While some runners plan on sixty-plus miles for training, in my mind that can lead to injuries and exhaustion.

Experiment with what works for you, and find your core running regimen, as we are all different and have different goals.

If I can hit four hours, give or take, in any marathon, I'm happy with my performance. Know what you really want and plan accordingly. My days of hoping to reach what was my personal best of 3:25 are probably over, based on what I know about my body today.

In New York, there are many different courses to test your training schedule. One of my favorites is to leave Central Park at Columbus Circle and head over to the running (and biking) trail that runs along the Hudson river. Sometimes I head north to the George Washington Bridge and do a turnaround, and sometimes I head south down to the Wall Street area. Both courses are filled with runners of all types and give anyone a smorgasbord of sights from the huge cruise ships at the piers to watching the sailboats on the river. You'll pass the various architectural wonders of the city, taking in the new Hudson Yards and more. The entire stretch is called the Greenway and runs from Battery Park up to 181st Street.

For those who prefer the East Side, the East River running path goes from the tip of Manhattan in Battery Park and is traffic-free for 4.5 miles to East 34th Street. Further north, start a run at East 84th Street in Carl Schurz Park and head north to 125th Street.

Generally, it's wise to stay off the main avenues when running in the city, as it's a maze of people, bicyclists, cars, and trucks. But with so many options along the rivers or in the city's parks, it's easy to plot out your desired course.

For the more intrepid runner who likes to shake it up a bit, take a run across the Brooklyn Bridge or hop on the subway to the 1,146-acre Van Cortlandt Park or the Pelham Bay Park, both in the Bronx. Pelham is New York's largest park at 2,765 acres and has great historical significance, playing a role in the American Revolution.

Some friends and I have a plan in the works to run in every major park in all five boroughs. We would add the Greenbelt in Staten Island, Flushing Meadow in Queens, and Prospect Park in Brooklyn. One of our ideas is to take 26.2 miles and divide it by 5 for 5.24 miles in each borough to create our own customized park marathon!

One solution may not work, so try a different one. If your life has fallen into a rut, change up your schedule to avoid stagnating. Try something new.

In the far stretches of Brooklyn, the Coney Island Boardwalk is a five-mile beachfront run that allows you to not only take in the sights, but has amazing peoplewatching and great food stalls for a post-run snack.

Like many cities, New York has all types of running clubs, from the well-known Central Park Track Club to the Boogie Down Bronx Runners. You can join the LGBT Front Runners group or a neighborhood group like the Crown Heights Running Club. Or you can start your own club. All it takes is an idea and a group of like-minded runners to make it happen. The granddaddy of them all is the New York Road Runners Club that not only oversees the NYC Marathon, but sponsors tons of races, seminars, club member benefits, and has a Club Council that helps the more than one hundred clubs in New York alone!

While New York is my hometown, how can you explore your city? What different courses can you run? How can you explore new neighborhoods and trails?

Every city has them. During a half marathon in Albuquerque, I discovered an amazing set of trails on the course. Try new routes to shake up your regimen. It'll make you more excited about your runs, and it's fun to discover new things.

One of my favorite discoveries was when a friend took me up to Runyon Canyon Park with amazing views of Los Angeles below. Most of my runs in that city had been along the ocean in Santa Monica or through Beverly Hills on Santa Monica Boulevard, but now I have a new place to go when I'm there.

For cities to which I travel on a regular basis, I try to develop at least three or four routes that I run when I go there. It lets me keep track of what is happening in the different neighborhoods over time.

On any given day in New York, you'll see runners everywhere, either by themselves or in small groups, a mother running and pushing her child's stroller or a father running with his kids. It's a running city at all times of the day.

Like many others, I'm also an all-weather runner. A snowstorm? No problem. One glorious morning when Central Park was a winter wonderland from an overnight snowfall, I was out and counted maybe a dozen other runners that braved the weather, including my friend Lindsay, who was enjoying the white silence that surrounded us. I'll never forget the beauty of that morning. I'm happy to run in rain or in heat but avoid lightning and thunderstorms or when it starts hitting ninety degrees. For me, any excuse to avoid treadmills is a good thing, as I need to feel the air and the wind and the smells of the environment around me.

Every New Yorker at one time or another fantasizes about running the New York City Marathon. It's one of the premier events in the world!

It all started in 1970, and all 26.2 miles were run in Central Park. The 127 entrants paid $1 to enter, but only 55 men finished, and the sole female entrant dropped out due to an illness. It wasn't until 1976 when the first five-borough run took place with 2,000 runners in the inaugural event.

According to George Hirsch, one of the founders of the event, it grew quickly. By 1978, there were 8,588 runners, and of course, today, it's one of the largest races in the world with 52,000 finishers in 2018! Throughout the years, many running records have been broken and milestones created in the New York marathon. A simple Google search will outline all of them for you.

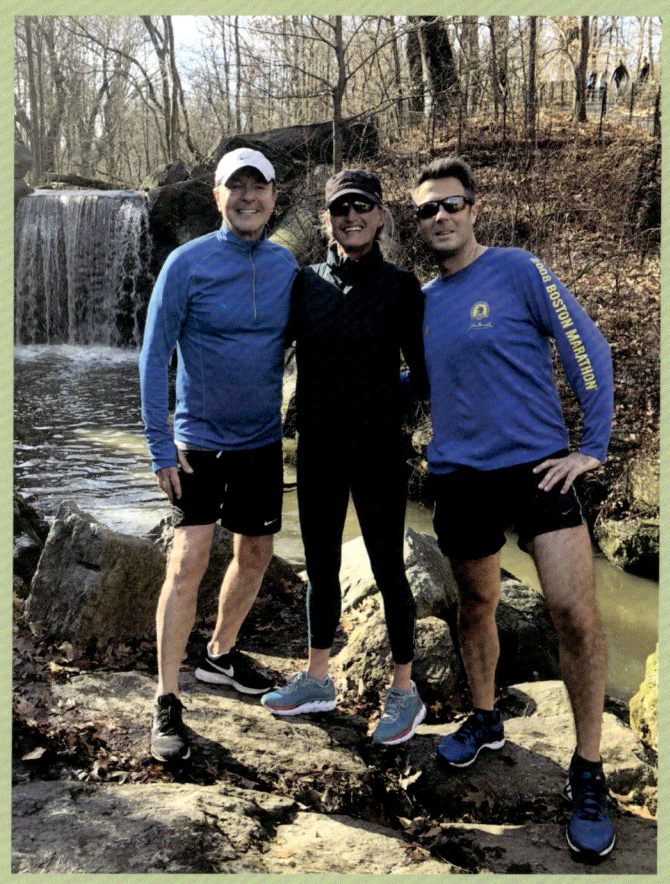

For me, any excuse to avoid treadmills is a good thing, as I need to feel the air and the wind and the smells of the environment around me.

It was never my intent to run a marathon, but like many, I got swept up in the idea of my hometown race and committed to learning what I had to do to train for the run.

While most of my focus has been on identifying marathons around the world to combine them with a travel experience, New York always beckons. My last New York City Marathon was in 2017, and it reminded me of the great glory of the race.

Starting in Staten Island at the base of the Verrazano Bridge is epic. The course, which runs through Brooklyn and Queens, lets me experience parts of the city I would never see. The explosive sight and sound of the spectators as you come off the Fifty-ninth Street bridge to run up First Avenue is one of the biggest rushes that any runner will ever experience. Heading north into the Bronx and then down Fifth Avenue to enter Central Park is a time of great anticipation and excitement as you get to the homestretch.

When I enter the park, I'm on my hometown turf again, and the last three miles of the race is as familiar to me as anything. It's where I spend hours and hours running for fun and training for a run, often times alone or with friends or my dog, Hannah.

For anyone who has never run a marathon, but has the hidden desire, New York will never disappoint. It will be one of your life's top moments that you'll never forget.

When I'm asked about my five best running experiences, completing my first marathon in New York City has to be one of them. The others would include running my first 10k; sharing my sister's first marathon finish in London; completing seven marathons on seven continents, with Antarctica being the climactic experience; and taking my nephew, Nicolas, out for his first run in Central Park. But there are many more that could fill its own chapter, including running in the wild in Tanzania; running the trails above Santa Fe; along the Seine in Paris; through the vineyards of Mendoza, Argentina; on Bondi Beach in Sydney; and in the early morning mist along the Bund in Shanghai.

What are your favorite running moments? It can be as simple as running your first complete mile, something you thought you could never do, or it could be completing your first race with your best friend, regardless of it being a 5k fun run or an ultra-marathon. Running memories will fill your life in ways that will always fulfill you.

You may meet the love of your life on a running trail or have a revelation that alluded you or make a monumental life decision. Savor those moments, all brought to you by your running life.

SEE MICHAEL'S FRIENDS RUN

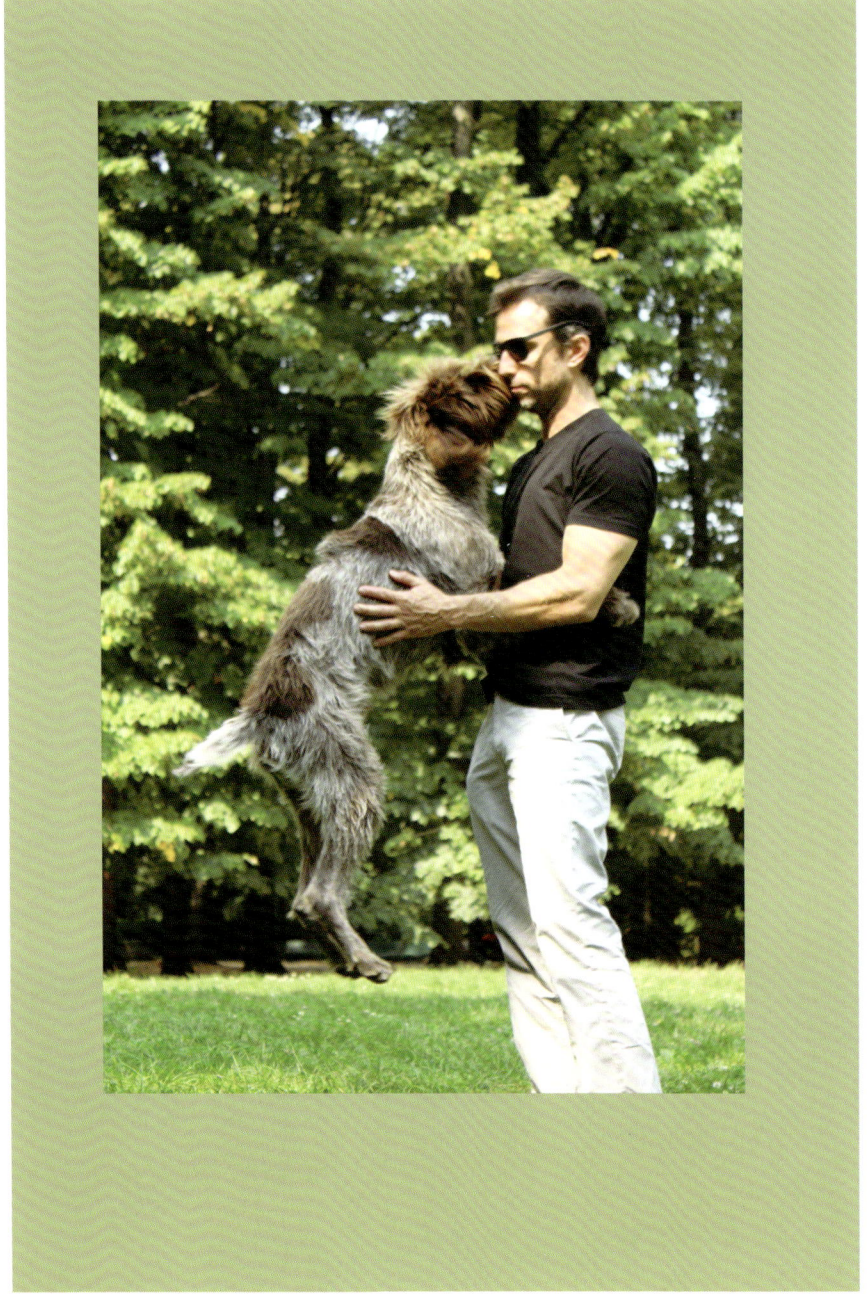

Running with the Dogs

Steve Sharp

In Los Angeles, there were two runs. To my north, four miles of sandstone bluffs, over manicured grass, gravel paths, and under palms. To my south, five miles of sand, level and firm as the ocean would make its retreat.

Then I moved to New York. Again, two runs were found. First there was downtown: Solitary Sunday mornings. Quiet streets and closed shops. A feeling as though the city were mine alone. Then came Central Park. Joining that endless procession of runners at dusk. Darkening treetops framed by buildings brightening behind.

My childhood sports hero came to New York for a tournament every year for many years. In an interview, he once said that Central Park can teach you everything you need to know about life. At that time, I had not yet seen Central Park, but this stuck with me.

One day, after all those days of running, of running alone, of running to outrun myself, I got a dog, and the running changed. Gone were the sacred Sunday mornings, the evening vigils in Central Park, replaced by a hunting dog, a rope between us, and that dragged-across-concrete feeling.

Barley is a Wirehaired Pointing Griffon. This as a name sounds fancy, but as a dog is anything but. The American Kennel Club describes Wirehaired Pointing Griffons as the supreme gun dog, known to thrive in both extreme weather and extreme terrain, and with the endurance of a marathon runner. Perfect for the West Village.

That first Winter, living downtown, we ran as best we could, Barley and me. Terrorized squirrels in Washington Square Park. Outmaneuvered park cops along the Hudson River and angry parents in sad city playgrounds. Until one day, I heard mention of off-leash hours every early morning at Central Park. And so it was, on that very next Saturday, a fine spring morning, a man and his supreme gun dog arose at first light, and leaving downtown for uptown, a new world opened before them.

If someone just came upon Central Park, I suppose they would assume that it's a bit of Manhattan island preserved. But having read just a little of its history, I knew the opposite was so. Fifteen years and the labor of thousands turned rock and swamp into the artistic vision of two men. A vision of varied scenes, a collection of canvases. Some in harmony, some in discord.

I won't ever forget that first morning when, together, Barley and I came upon Central Park. I'd never seen it under an early morning light. Standing on Umpire Rock, two kings looking for a Kingdom. Fleeing an Egypt behind us to conquer a Jericho before us. Following Barley, I would break free from the unbroken chain of runners. An endless circle trapped within a rectangle. Asphalt would be traded for grass and rocks and streams. The rhythmic shuffling of feet would be replaced by racing and jumping and stopping and looking. The known would be tossed aside for just a little bit of unknown.

One day, after all those days of running, of running alone, of running to outrun myself, I got a dog, and the running changed.

First, past a placid Shakespeare, Sir Walter and Robbie Burns, we ran into The Mall. Under its cathedral ceiling of American elms, with Barley racing over green lawns. Crashing down stairs, and for a moment into darkness, but under a glittering ceiling, then out and onto that sanctuary of open sky, Bethesda Terrace, where tourists laughed, and the Angel of Waters disapproved as Barley dove into her baptismal font.

Then to The Lake, smooth as stone, and along its north shore, deep coves encircled by The Rambles. Racing over Bow Bridge and lost into that landscape. A mystery of twisted and tangled forest, with its labyrinth of paths, of stairways and steps carved into broken bedrock. Now running upstream, emptying from an unknown above, and at last breaking free and onto Vista Rock, with a towering castle beside us, and lifting Barley so he can catch his own glimpse of The Great Lawn awaiting below.

Now racing under cherry trees, bare and brown, and beyond the North Meadow to The Pool. Dark water on that morning but a deep bed of bright green on so many other. Following this same water as it emptied into a ravine. Jumping down steps of bedrock. Under a stone arch, around a bend, and lost into a forest of streams and stones and swamps. A great fallen tree. A single duck moving over thin water. But then aflight, as Barley crashed into The Loch.

South now and running for home. Across the slope of Cedar Hill. Perfectly graded for summer reading and winter sledding. But at all mornings of all seasons somehow perfect, too, as the city's biggest congregation of dogs and dog-owners. Both of all shapes and sizes, but impossibly all of only one mood: friendly, maybe even happy. Despite the harsh reminder of the city still resting in plain view.

From that first morning, and on the many mornings after, I have seen all that Central Park has to offer. Time and time again. Yet on every morning run, every time, the lessons keep on coming. Like a great art gallery, where there is something new to discover, something new to learn, each time you go.

But I know that without Barley, I would not have learned these lessons. As I know that without Barley, I would still be running the same. Running to outrun myself. Running along the path well-traveled.

Maybe Central Park really can teach you everything there is to know about life. But for me, the real lesson was found in running with a dog.

Steve Sharp *is a media executive. Barley is a squirrel executive. Together, they've run in parks from Milan to Toronto to Monaco. But they're both happiest on sunny Saturday mornings in Central Park.*

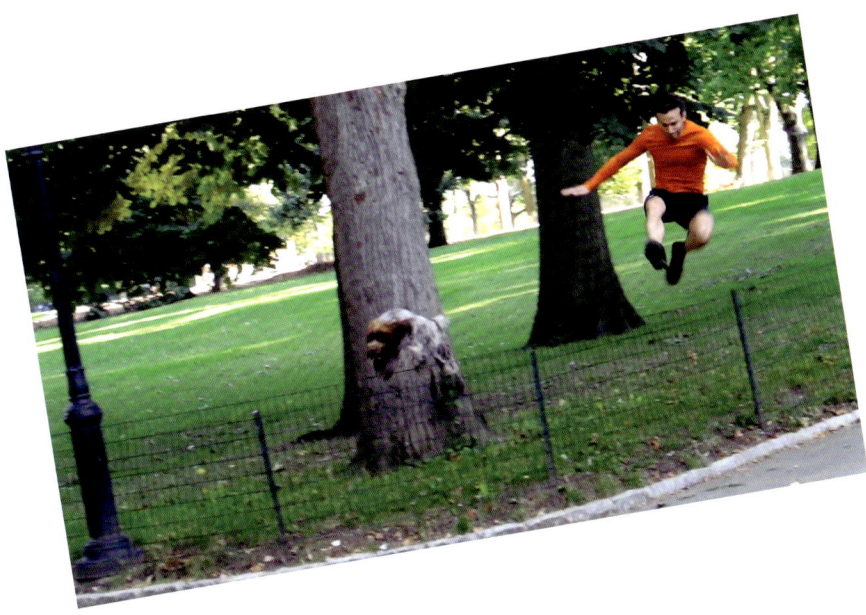

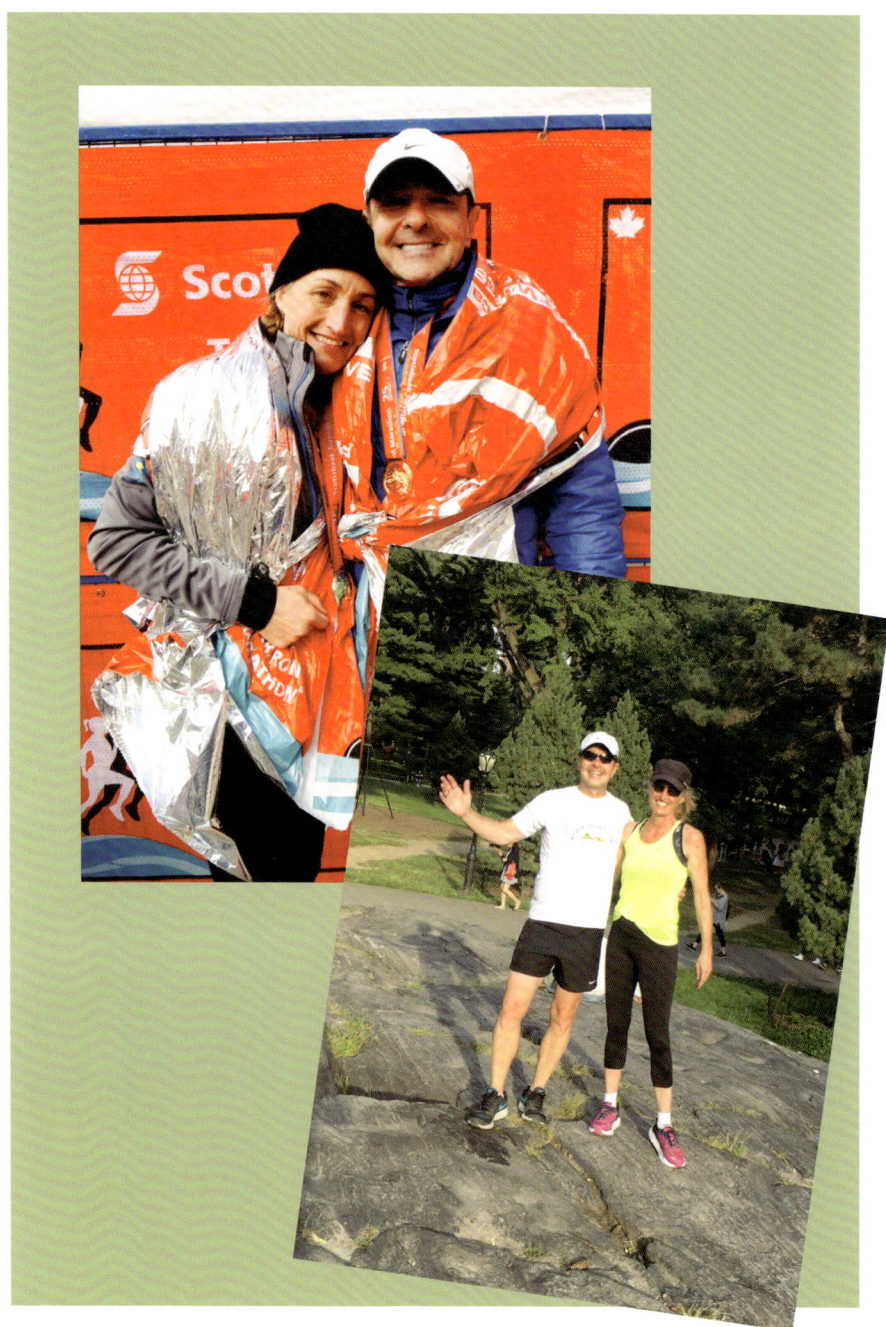

Meditation Movement

Emily Mingenbach-Henry

My love for running started in college when a friend, Kimberly, took me out for a jog. It was short, only about two miles. Even so, I was hit with such a remarkable running high that I knew I had found my medicine. That expansive sensation, that lift of spirit, that feeling of being one with the universe was coursing through me on that very first run. The following day, my legs felt like they had been beaten with a baseball bat, but nothing could have stopped me from putting on those shoes and doing it again.

From then on, the mysticism and spirituality of running has guided me through life. I started things off with a bang in my early running days. I returned to Taos after college to ski and play for a few years. I started to run out on the pueblo land behind my house with my parents' three dogs. It wasn't exactly legal for me to be out there, but I did it anyway. I feel compelled to write, somewhat defensively and immaturely, that lots of "whiteys" trespassed onto Indian land back then. I mean, no one seemed to be out there, anyway. Besides, a running buddy from the Pueblo always used to encourage me to run there and insisted that it really was okay. This made me feel special and unique and deeply entitled to trespass. Even so, every once in a while, I would be chased down by a scowling man on a horse and told to get off Indian land immediately. I would sadly turn around and do the run of shame back home.

But I would keep going back. Believe me, it was a powerful force that lured me deeper and deeper into those mountains. I even found running gear the color of the trees and shrubs to wear for camouflage. My heart would beat faster knowing I was doing something I shouldn't do. The thrill of sneaking up there undetected was addictive. I couldn't stop myself from heading east into those mountains.

Then some things started happening. Starting small, I almost stepped on a rattler. Two times. Well, that's no big deal, I told myself—I mean, it's a big deal if you get a snakebite, but I was spared, so all good, right?

I want to back up and explain that the dogs were my alarms. For the duration of the runs, they would circle me. When nothing was amiss, I hardly saw them. But if all three were with me, I always knew that something was wrong. They would never bark (they were too smart for that); instead, they would just hover up close to me, alerting me to danger. One day, I was going up a sandy wash at the base of the mountains and—*bam*—all three dogs were right under me. Hm . . . Then I got a creepy feeling, a feeling of being watched or tracked. The dogs started whining softly. Not good. I turned around and headed back down. Something was terribly wrong. And it was just then that I looked down and saw huge mountain lion tracks covering our tracks going up. I panicked. Of course, I did exactly what they say NOT to do: I put it into high gear and ran as fast as I could out of those woods and down onto the alluvial plain, where I could see my house in the distance.

In short order, I took a break from going up there for a few weeks while I thought about that big cat and how it silently watched and followed us. If it had wanted to hurt us, it certainly could have. Instead, with all that power and strength, it let us be. I wondered if one of my spirit animals might be a mountain lion. Probably not, but I bought a small lion fetish and put it on my altar, anyway. Eventually I decided it was a mystical experience full of wonder, showing me there is much more to this world than what we see, smell, and touch.

In short order, I was back to my old tricks and started going even farther than before. One day, we got to one of our new spots up on the mountain that I appreciated because of the view. It's an unusual place because it has no trees and is relatively flat. I could stop and look out across Taos Ski Valley all the way up into Colorado. This particular day, we reached the clearing and all of a sudden, out of nowhere, five coyotes surrounded us. In an instant, three coyotes attacked the three dogs and two more were staring me down, snarling. I grabbed rocks and sticks, I hooted and hollered and finally got the coyotes away from the dogs and me. We managed to get down after the harrowing decent. The dogs were cut up and bloody, a couple needed stitches. It's very unusual to be attacked like that; coyotes usually keep to themselves and have no use for trouble of that sort. Whatever the reason, they definitively made it clear we were out of bounds. I never went back to that place. The universe had spoken: I was not supposed to be there.

If you can believe it, I still continued to take the dogs up onto pueblo land, although on a shorter route. That is, until this next occurrence: toward the end of that summer, the dogs and I had done a small loop and were heading back down. It was a bright, clear sunny morning, and we were on the alluvial plain with nothing but low sagebrush around us. We were about a mile from home when I heard a loud clap just to my left. Curious. Nothing there. Fifty yards down, another loud clap just on my left. Nothing there. By this point, my fear factor is registering super high. This was not explainable. And finally, after another hundred yards or so, another loud clap to my left. The mountain lion was scary and so were the coyotes, but this situation frightened me the most because these sounds came from another world. That was the end. I finally decided never to go back there again.

A while later, I bumped into my running buddy from the pueblo at the Taos Inn. He asked how the running was going, and I proceeded to tell him about the mountain lion, the coyotes, and, finally, the mysterious clapping sound. While I was recounting my story, his face started to change. By the end, he looked alarmed. He was quiet for some time, and he looked at me with the most serious face, full of concern and worry, and said, "Emily, I believe you must never step foot up there ever again." And he got up and left. I knew better than to expect an explanation; for good reason, Native Americans, particularly those at Taos Pueblo, are extremely secretive about their culture, traditions, and religion. But I did hear one thing of note a few years later: someone told my mother that the witches of the pueblo gather on that clearing and that they can transform into coyotes to avoid being seen.

Eventually I decided it was a mystical experience full of wonder, showing me there is much more to this world than what we see, smell, and touch.

I mourned the loss of my spirit place, but I knew that I was no longer welcome there. Was I ever welcome? I had always thought so: as a child, I spent days there riding my little Yamaha 60, collecting arrowheads and potsherds. I had grown up thinking it was my backyard. But that was then and things change. This time, the message was that I had invaded some spirit world that wasn't expecting my company. For thirty years, I have never gone up onto Indian land again. I will continue to respect their wishes, whoever or whatever "they" are. Those experiences were humming with danger and tinged with darkness. Regardless, that was when I was introduced to the world of trail running, the freedom we experience along with the risks we take out in those mountains. No longer an innocent, I had been seduced by the wilds.

Leaving those mystical experiences behind, it's time to write about a spiritual path that is more pragmatic, practical, and long lasting—and less dangerous, might I add. Still, whether it's mystical or spiritual, or both, my point is that running helps me jump into that fourth dimension, where time and space become irrelevant and I can join, even if for just nanoseconds, the Great Positive Energy Field.

Challenges or triumphs, running gives me space to observe and rejoice all that is handed me. Often the problems du jour are silly ones—ones that I can't remember having the next week. Others have been deep wounds, excavated out of my soul by the simple action of lacing up a pair of shoes and heading out the door. Day after day, week after week, year after year, my spiritual experience grows. The beauty is that it knows no bounds. So, how free do I want to be? It's up to me.

I'm not a religious person but am a deeply spiritual one. In my view, meditation and prayer are essential to a happy, healthy, and productive life. As much as I try, meditation and prayer are very difficult for me when I'm sitting still. But when I run, it's like a portal is opened to the mystery of the universe. Tapping into that positive energy is an immense gift, and I am grateful that I understand the true nature of my problems (spiritual) and have the solution (at my feet, if you will) to help me. I have come to understand that no amount of self-will can help with my problems. If I am facing down something overwhelming at work, let's say, it's not advisable to forgo my run to get to the office early so I can get to my desk and panic; that will be less productive and less instructive than starting the day with prayer and meditation through a run. I compare this concept to the Pleiades, a constellation that's so faint it's only visible by shifting your gaze off to the side. When you look straight at it, it disappears. Running offers insight by clearing my mind so there's space for God to show me what really is important.

On a normal six-mile run, my typical experience goes something like this:

Mile one: Chatter. Committee in session. Negative thinking. Bickering. Disputes. Grievances.

Mile two: Less chatter. Half of the committee has abandoned their posts and left for the day. Prayers creep in. Brief relapses into negativity and bickering. Remaining committee members no longer interested in my problems. Move back into prayer.

Mile three: A voice says, "Let go." My body relaxes. Hey! I don't remember running up the big hill. How am I already here?

Mile Four: Wow. It's really beautiful out here. I'm so grateful.

Mile Five: Something tells me to consider honesty, hope, and faith. I ponder that for a while. (This is often when some sort of mystical thing happens: a family of magpies follows me and my dog for a long time, "talking" to us.)

Mile six: Everything melted away. I am deeply connected to the positive potentiality of the universe. Look at that, I'm home.

Running is the ultimate spiritual reset button. After a run, my mind is sharp, my thoughts are clear, and my moral compass seems fortified. Connecting with something bigger diminishes my fear. Less afraid, I'm less likely to make decisions based on fear that can hurt others or me. I can instead act with love and kindness and I can remember my responsibility to be respectful of others. Why running does this for me is a great mystery, but I don't worry about the why. There's a great saying that goes something like this: "If I can imagine it, it is not God."

As a rule, I run solo with my dog. The only exception is Michael (the author of this book). Therefore, it should not be a surprise that I have very mixed feelings about races. No doubt, marathons are incredible accomplishments. The discipline to train for one is intense, and the dedication to make it over the finish line is huge. But I will always prefer to run alone, with the God of my understanding as my running mate.

The first marathon I did was in Toronto on my forty-fifth birthday. My marriage had fallen apart. Par for the course, the separation was rough. Michael called me and said, ". . . this is what you are going to do, missy. You are going to run this marathon with us . . ." He emailed me a training spreadsheet and generously bought me a roundtrip ticket (I was broke at the time), and I hit the trails and ran my way through one of the hardest chapters of my life.

Training schedules are time consuming, especially those last six weeks leading up to the race. As the runs got longer, my focus became narrower: work, kids, and run. I retreated from many of the old distractions of life. I suppose some could see this as isolation, but it didn't feel that way at all. Profound feelings of loss and failure coupled with a crushing fear of the future made it difficult to keep from spinning out. That feeling of impending doom was on call 24/7. Thankfully, running has always offered freedom from myself, a respite to just exist in the moment so I can connect to something bigger (and far more comforting) than my own thoughts. Training forced me to simplify my life. In exchange for four pairs of worn out Hokas, I received a powerful dose of self-love, gratitude, and forgiveness. What a bargain. Michael's plan was a godsend.

I pushed myself to the edge, running fourteen-plus milers from seven thousand to eleven thousand feet and back. Many of those runs were solid crying from start to finish, snot and all. I laugh, imagining what I looked like running through the Santa Fe Forest looking so tragic. The few unfortunates I came across looked stricken with concern when they saw me. I had to promise them that I really was okay. In the end, everyone understands heartbreak. I discovered my limits and learned acceptance. This process, this therapy for my soul, was equal parts pain and healing. Crying and running, running and crying, I made it through. Once again, the spirituality of running saved me.

Running and finishing the Berlin Marathon was and will always be one of the highlights of my life. Zigzagging through that mysterious city (that I had never visited before) past 26.2 miles of cheering onlookers was magical, with that spectacular finish under the Brandenburg Gate and into the Tiergarten. It was one of the most incredible four hours of my life.

I will preemptively apologize for what I'm about to say next, as I'm pretty sure that I'm about to contradict many of the other essays in this book—all I'm doing here is writing my personal experience. The mundane aspects of races don't appeal to me. Crowds make me uncomfortable. The pre-race noise, confusion, and hype give me negative anxiety. The joy of running is diminished when I'm surrounded by thousands of hyper people so excited to prove themselves at the starting gate of a race. Please believe that I honor any person running a race and I don't judge anyone's motives. Races are wonderful things. But still, it's not my snapshot of a great time. I have been stuck in a pack of people who are breathing as loud as hippos, spitting and moaning, sometimes vomiting and passing out, and it strips all the grace and dignity away from this otherwise elegant and classy sport.

I'm sure it's very different for the running elite and the super-fast runners who are way ahead of the foaming pack of yahoos, but I'm often stuck smack dab in the mediocre runners, especially at the beginning. By the middle of the race, everyone spreads out and I start gaining on the enthusiastic starters who are losing steam. By the last third, I'm consistently gaining on people and I'm mentally wrestling to find some sort of bright side about running in the race. It would be a stretch to call it a spiritual experience.

The last race I did was in Albuquerque. I finished. It was fine. We ended up having fun that day, but I could have done without the race. It lacked the luster of some of the other races I've participated in. I have decided to give myself permission to stop racing for a while. Time will tell. I might be back at it sooner than I think.

But I will always prefer the hinterlands, when I'm alone with my dog and all is quiet and serene both inside and outside. Where the air is fragrant, the ground is soft, and the mountains are singing beautiful lullabies through the trees. And the universe can whisper sweet nothings into my soul. Or, perhaps, send a pack of coyotes to teach me a much-needed lesson.

Emily Mingenbach-Henry *lives in Santa Fe, New Mexico. She has been running the mountains of northern New Mexico for more than thirty years.*

Diplomacy on the Run

Amir Arasta

The first time I heard about the Persian Gulf Marathon in Iran was in 2016. I received an email that indicated that there would be a 40-kilometer marathon from Shiraz to the 2,500-year-old historical ruin, Persepolis. My excitement quickly turned into suspicion, however, as the website for the marathon was European-based, rather than Iranian, and asking for euro as a form of payment. As much as I wanted to participate in the race, I passed.

A few months after that, on the day of the race, my mother called me from Iran and told me she was watching the race on TV. After checking the website and seeing the pictures, a part of me was very happy that the race was successfully held in Iran and another part of me was very unhappy that I missed it!

A year later, once again I received an email about the second marathon in Iran, which was going to be held in Tehran this time. It has always been my dream to run a marathon in my birthplace. After some searching on the internet and a few emails, I convinced myself to sign up. After all, if the race was cancelled, I could use my time visiting family and sightseeing.

I decided to wear a green shirt with IRAN written on the front, a pair of white shorts, and red socks to represent my nationality, heart, and soul. But I could not just consider my roots without my branches and leaves. So, I decided to wear an American flag to show my gratitude and appreciation toward the country that helped me achieve my goals and dreams.

In March 2017, I booked a trip to Tabriz in northern Iran for few days of sightseeing before heading to Tehran. As I was flying from Tabriz to Tehran, I saw an advertisement in the newspaper about the race. That was the moment I realized it was really going to happen. It was a two-loop race, and it would start in Iran's biggest stadium, Azadi Stadium, and end in Azadi Square, ten kilometers away. I had been in that stadium more than fifty times to attend soccer games, so it was very exciting for me to run a marathon there.

On the morning of the race, I had someone come pick me up and take me straight to the stadium. It was Friday, and thankfully the weather promised to be sunny. There

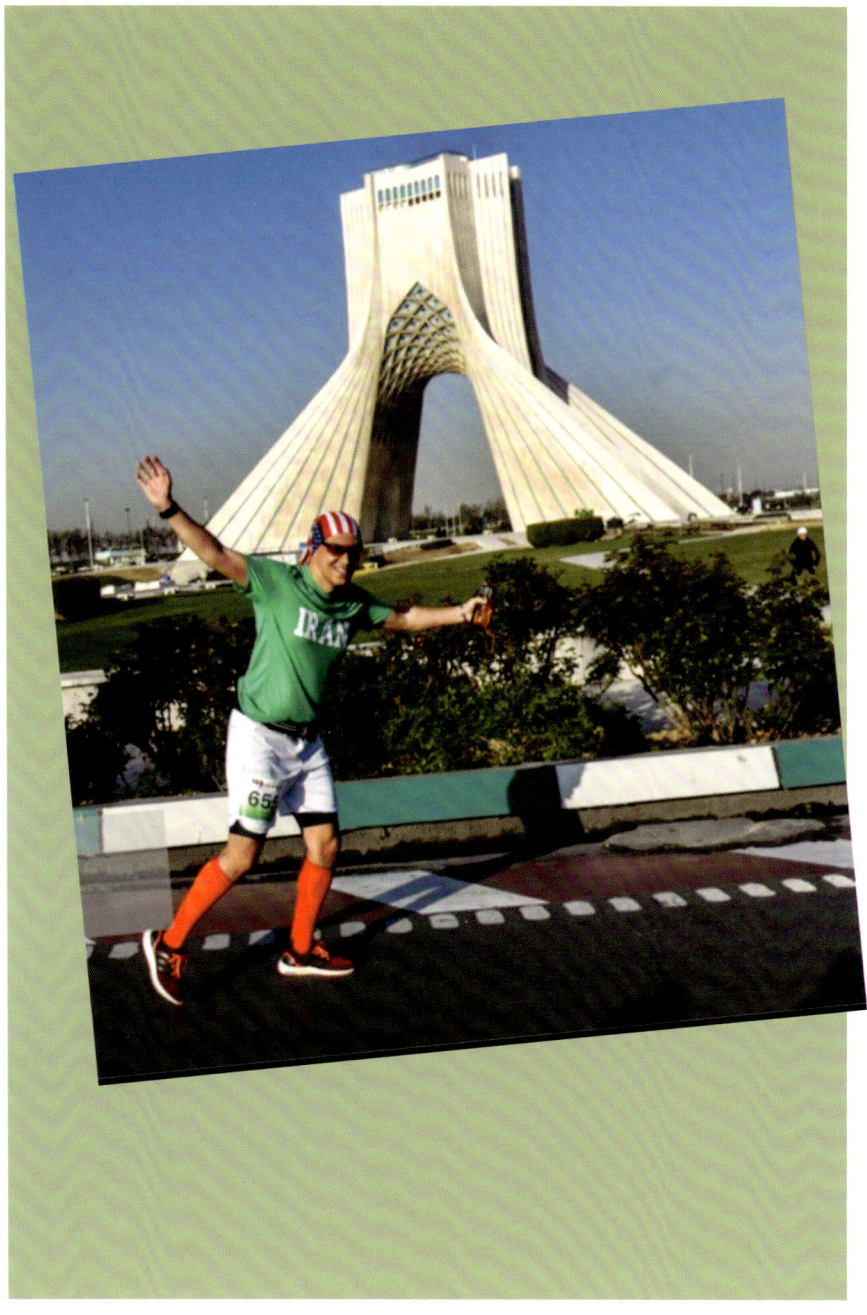

are days in Tehran when the pollution is high due to traffic, but Fridays are usually better since the traffic is lighter than normal. When we got to the stadium, we were instructed to go to a building to change our clothes.

After I changed into my running clothes, I put my US flag bandana on and walked out of the building. As soon as I walked out, I thought maybe wearing a US bandana wasn't a good idea. Everybody was looking at me like I was naked. I had two options: go back to the building and take the bandana off or look back at them as if *they're naked*! I decided on the second option and started to warm up and stretch. After a few minutes, some runners from Japan came up to take a picture with me, and very soon I became "the guy we should take a picture with!"

I decided to wear a green shirt with IRAN written on the front, a pair of white shorts, and red socks to represent my nationality, heart, and soul.

I ended up taking pictures with many people who assumed I was an American. They seemed surprised that I wanted to run with an American flag on the streets of Tehran. Later, I learned that all the American and English runners were not able to get visas to come to Iran. In the middle of picture-taking, reporters from different news agencies in and outside of Iran held microphones in front of me and asked me who I was and where I came from. Some assumed I was an American and started speaking English before I told them I was Iranian. From the corner of my eyes, I could see that the minister of sport was also surrounded by reporters. A reporter came up to me and said he was from the national TV station and would like to film me, but I had to remove the bandana in order for it to air. When I said no, he walked away, disappointed.

The race started almost on time, and I was very impressed about the way they closed the roads and with the level of security and police enforcement. Tehran is a very big city, and the event is in the middle of the town, so blocking off the traffic takes an army! As I neared Azadi Square, I saw that some people were waiting and cheering for runners. As soon as they noticed me, they started pointing me out to the others and screaming "America! America!" For most of them, I was the only American they had ever seen in real life.

As I was running around Azadi Square, heading back to Azadi Stadium, I heard a vehicle coming up from behind me, and someone was saying, "Pull over, pull over!" Knowing that the roads were closed to people, I thought the vehicle must belong to the authorities. I knew there was a high risk that the vehicle belonged to government officials or the special police who would want me to stop and go to the side of the road to question my identity and the reason I was wearing a US flag bandana. I did not turn my head back to look; I pretended I didn't understand what the guy was saying and kept running.

The vehicle drove up on my right side, and I turned my head to look at it. It was a van with about ten or twelve reporters and photographers trying to tell the driver to pull over to get closer to me so that they could take my picture! They kept asking me to look this way and that way to take pictures like I was a celebrity. As I got back to the stadium, finishing my first loop, I could sense that people were waking up in Tehran and crowds were starting to gather. I found two other Iranians who asked me if they could join me on the second loop. One was doing his second marathon after finishing his first in Paris, and the other one was a teenager doing his first marathon. I might be wrong, but I had a feeling they wanted to protect me in case something happened to me.

As soon as they noticed me, they started pointing me out to the others and screaming "America! America!"

On the second loop, I got some high-fives from people saying: "Go America!" or "Yes!" I also heard two or three people expressing their disapproval upon seeing my bandana and questioning my presence in Iran. I pretended not to understand, although my Farsi is perfect, and just kept running. I let my running companions respond to them, telling them to leave me alone, explaining that I was Iranian. But mostly people were confused about my clothes, representing the Iranian flag and the name of Iran on my chest while also wearing the American flag.

By the time I was heading back to the stadium for the second time to finish the race, I was pretty tired. About half a mile to the stadium, I met my friends and family, and one of my running companions recognized my cousin, surprising us all. What a small world. After passing the finish line, there were more people who wanted to take a picture with me before I headed back to the locker room to change. I took some pictures with two attendants who were watching our clothes for us. The best part was when the two guys asked the security guard with a walkie-talkie to join us and he refused by saying: "I will lose my job taking a picture with an American!" Even when I told him in Farsi that I was a native Iranian, he said the flag was a problem.

After the race, I went home and checked my phone. I had some messages from friends in the United States saying that they had seen me all over the Farsi language sites running with an American bandana and asking me if I was crazy. Some told me to

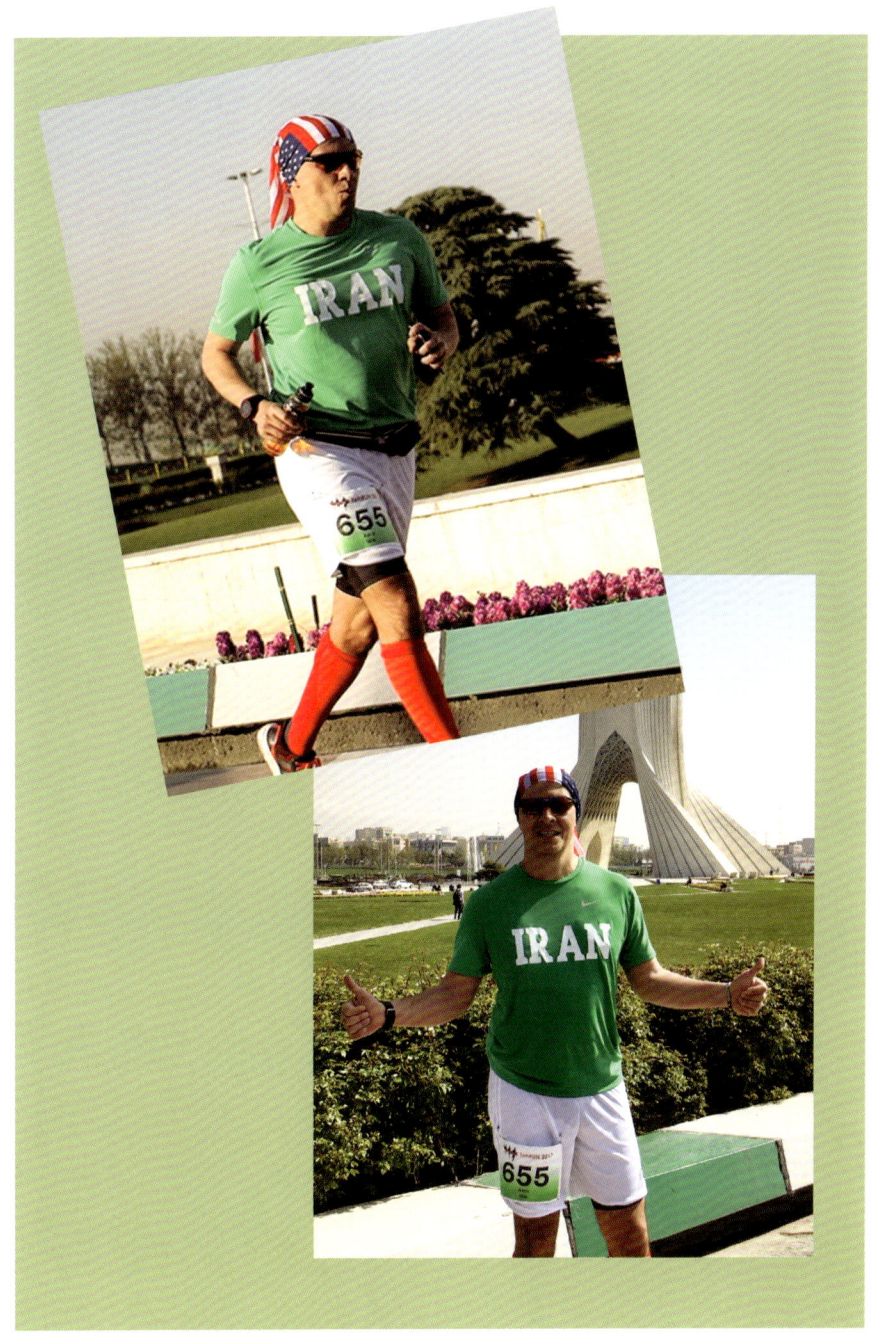

leave before they figure out who I was and arrest me. That evening, a program on TV talked about the first marathon in Tehran, and one of the reporters asked if Americans traveled to Iran for the race, and the presenter said unfortunately they could not get the visas on time and that there was only one person with dual citizenship, an Iranian American, who ran the race. A few days later, I left Tehran with the finisher's medal close to my heart in my pocket without any problem.

> *But mostly people were confused about my clothes, representing the Iranian flag and the name of Iran on my chest while also wearing the American flag.*

When I got back to the United States, I received an email from the guy who put the whole race together, thanking me for coming to Iran to participate in the race. He is Dutch, married to an Iranian, and lives in Iran. He said I represented what the race was all about: creating a bridge between the nations. After a few emails between us, I realized how hard it was for him to put everything together and that he was doubting if he could ever do it again. But he did, as the Persian Gulf Marathon took place on the island of Kish in early 2019.

I've run over fifty-five marathons, but that day in Tehran will be the one that stays with me forever as I expressed both my Iranian heritage and my American life on the city's streets.

Amir Arasta *has run more than fifty-five marathons, including on all seven continents, five majors, and forty states. He also finished an IRONMAN last year. His goal is running one hundred marathons and six IRONMANs in six continents.*

Running Through Life

Jean Chatzky

I started running my first fall in a new hometown on what felt like a dare, or maybe an admonishment. Back from a summer away, about to start my sophomore year at a high school in the new town my family had moved to over the summer, I had put on a few pounds. At a welcome-to-the-neighborhood barbeque, a couple of girls my age mentioned they were joining the cross-country track team. "Maybe you should do that, too, it would be a good way to meet people," she said. "And get back into shape," I heard.

But I didn't have any other after-school activities, so I joined. It was, I realize now, my first team of any sort. My first sport. There had been no soccer, no field hockey or lacrosse, certainly no gymnastics for me. I had tried out for cheerleading once with laughable results, the inability to do a cartwheel much less a split a bright dividing line between me and the girls chosen to don the uniform.

Cross-country was different. For practice, we just ran, sometimes three miles—mimicking the length of our races—sometimes up to ten. There were days we hit the track to do speed work, which I hated. The meets, for me, were the worst part. I consistently came in closer to last than first. (The one victory I hold onto was on a bus trip to a meet three hours away. I was the last one standing in an all-team match of the card game Screw Your Neighbor.) On the course, I always finished. And I learned that finishing counted, because we often needed my scores for the team to qualify. But mostly, we practiced—bunching into smaller groups and doing something that simply felt like going for a run. We talked, laughed, gossiped. And my father was right about one thing in particular: I did meet people. More than that, I made friends. On the night before high school graduation, as I looked around the group I was hanging with—girls and boys—most, I realized, were from that team.

And so began a pattern. When I packed up for college, I took running shoes with me. They didn't—admittedly—see a lot of daylight during those four years, but as I moved to New York City after graduation, they did. I found myself looking to connect with people I wanted to spend time with by suggesting that instead of drinks or dinner, maybe we should go on a run.

I met Gary through my roommate in Brooklyn. He was a few years older than me, worked in banking, lived on the Upper East Side, which made him a geographically undesirable running partner. But we shared an interest in cooking and Jewish music, and we both liked to run. So, several evenings a week, we made it work. I'd meet him at his apartment and we'd log four or five miles along the East River or, if we were up for the surprisingly steep incline from First Avenue to Central Park, run laps around the reservoir. What did we talk about? Whether Liz, the roommate who had introduced us, would marry Michael, her current boyfriend. (She did.) And whether Gary should join three of our other friends who were quitting their jobs to travel the world for six months. (He didn't.) In other words, everything—and nothing—as good running partners do.

I found myself looking to connect with people I wanted to spend time with by suggesting that instead of drinks or dinner, maybe we should go on a run.

Wally and I knew each other from a previous job and reconnected when we both joined the same magazine startup. Magazine startups, unlike the tech startups of today, had much less-demanding schedules, at least this one did. We were publishing every other month, which meant the bosses weren't showing up at the office every morning until close to ten. Wally and I figured we could do that, too, which is how we started running most mornings before work. I was living in Hell's Kitchen, so I'd enter Central Park at Columbus Circle and run up the East Side, picking her up at Seventy-Second Street. We'd continue together up and around the reservoir back around the west side. She'd drop me off where I began and finish the last mile on her own. All in all, I'd land at my desk with 5.2 miles under my belt and a toasted bialy with butter in my hands by 9:45.

I hatched my plans for life as a grown-up with Wally. I had been married a couple of years. The first ones weren't the easiest, but we'd settled in and were now thinking about kids, a move to the suburbs, what all of that meant for work, career, ambition. Wally was a wise, very slightly older sister, back in New York after her first marriage ended in divorce. I've tried therapy at several points during my life and quit, always thinking that I failed because I wasn't willing to go deep enough or give it the time it needed to succeed. Now, I think maybe I just didn't need it. I had a running partner instead.

When I created the wish list* of baby gifts I hoped to receive after giving birth for the first time, a baby jogger was at the top. (*Not an official registry. My mother was far

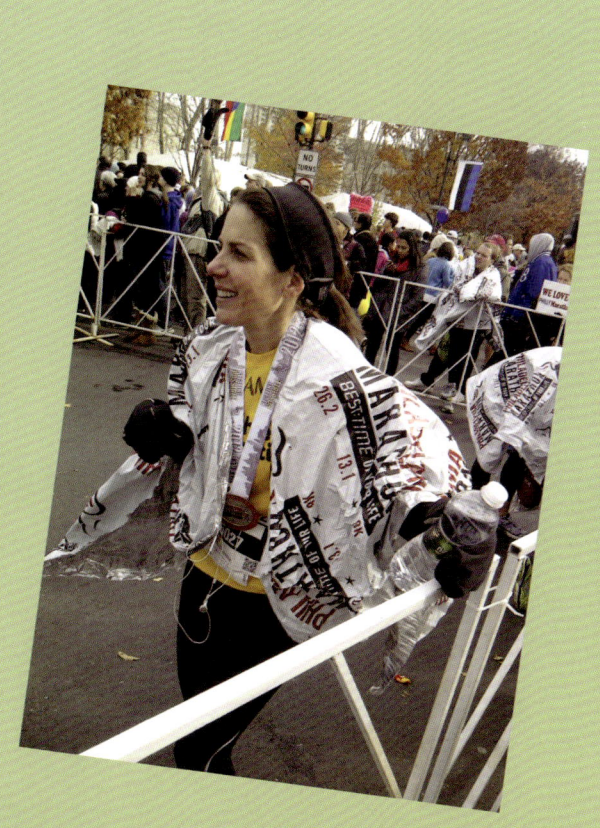

And so began a pattern. When I packed up for college, I took running shoes with me.

too superstitious to allow that.) Diane, my new neighbor in the suburbs, had one, too. She'd strap Ben into the jogger at her house, making sure to tuck a bottle into the back just in case, and I'd do the same with Jake at mine, and we'd meet in the middle on a street named Tuttle. It was conveniently divided by a grassy median and a half-mile from end to end, perfect for laps. Sometimes Gary, and his daughter Morgan, just about the same age as Jake, would drive over from his town about twenty minutes away and join us. But mostly it was just us two. When the boys outgrew the jogger, the girls—three years their junior, arriving a month apart—went in. And by the time the girls outgrew it, we were tired of pushing the damn things anyway. We just wanted to run.

> *And by the time the girls outgrew it,*
> *we were tired of pushing the damn things anyway.*
> *We just wanted to run.*

It has been more than two decades. The kids graduated high school and college. Diane and I have both lost our fathers. I've gotten divorced and remarried. She went back to school, got a master's degree, and found work that she loves. Today, Ben and Jake live a mile from each other in a city across the country. But still, we run. And lament when we can't. (As I write this, I'm getting over a bout of the flu. "Are you better yet?" Diane texted me this morning. "Yes, but not ready to run yet. Are you going without me?" I responded. "Nope," she said. "I'm getting on the elliptical. I need you to get me out of the house when it's this cold.")

I am now at the age and stage where my friends are moving once again. Diane and her husband are contemplating an apartment in Austin, closer to her mother. Other close friends have up and left for Florida, the city, Mexico. My husband and I are thinking about Philadelphia—near to my mother and the Jersey town where we spend weekends in the summer. My mother is worried that I won't have enough friends and that because I'm at an age where my children aren't there to bring us together, it'll be too difficult to make them.

But I know she's wrong. I'll find them on the run.

Jean Chatzky *has run one marathon and a half-dozen halves, but she prefers a good five-mile trail run with friends at a pace good for conversation. Off the trail, she's the financial editor of NBC Today, host of the HerMoney podcast, and financial ambassador for AARP.*

The Road to Recovery

Marc Metrick

My romance with running is a long and winding one, with several different ups and downs, sharp turns, drink breaks, and music. Not so different from a marathon . . .

I was in my mid-thirties when I met my first treadmill. I was having a successful career, albeit at the expense of almost everything else in my life. I was drinking too much, eating with reckless abandon, not sleeping a wink—altogether, not paying attention to "me" at all. It all changed one day in 2008. My boss, the company's chairman, came to see me. He let me know that the board of directors, and most of my colleagues, were getting concerned about my health. At 6 feet and 320 pounds, nobody was wrong. I needed to lose weight and change my lifestyle—and fast. The next day, I joined a gym and signed up with a personal trainer.

At first, it was grueling. The core body work was like learning a foreign language for my muscles. The treadmill was a welcome break; it offered a familiar friend in an otherwise new and scary sixty-minute training session. At my size, it was walking on an incline. See, walking wasn't new; it was comfortable. I had confidence when doing it. I kept going to the gym, started eating better, and lost a lot of weight—about seventy pounds. By then, I could run . . . well, maybe jog. Two or three days a week, three miles per run at a ten-minute pace, listening to music, while watching TV—oh, and treadmill only. After all, I told myself, "it's easier when the floor is moving at your pace."

My Tuesday and Thursday running schedule went on for another few months. I felt great on the treadmill and kept losing weight. I was making progress. My problem now shifted from my weight to the only caloric cheat on my new diet: alcohol.

See, I was always a heavy drinker, but I was able to handle myself. After all, at 320 pounds, you can drink a lot and keep going. Problem was, I was now tipping the scales at 250 and dropping fast. The booze caught up with me. I was eating healthier and running but drinking more than ever. The next few months are for another book, with another point, but in the end, I found myself in rehab in Malibu Beach, California. There I discovered the wonder of an outdoor run (they didn't have treadmills). I began to feel what running could be for me.

I started slow, literally. A nice ten-minute pace on the running path looking over the Pacific. I still listened to music, but now I was learning more about breathing, thinking about my gait, and focusing on the visual cues. I was only running two miles, but it was comforting to me to feel my distance at every quarter as I ran by familiar landmarks. Mostly, I enjoyed the solitude. The music was on my headphones, but I was coaching myself. I would say things like "half way to the half way mark." It became therapy for me. It was my release. It wasn't just the physical endorphin rush, but the feeling of accomplishment I'd have after the run. This was a time in my life that was dark and uncertain. I found running to be my comfort, my sense of security. It actually replaced the bottle. In those twenty-eight days in Malibu, I ran twice a day, two miles in the morning and one at night. Between my runs, I'd "do the work" as they say, focusing on my sobriety. Part of the work was becoming more introspective. So much so, meditation is actually one of the twelve steps in AA (step 11). But I struggled to meditate. I couldn't focus, couldn't relax my mind . . . I hit a block. Then I realized I do meditate; twice a day when I'm on my run. I had never known the sensation of being completely in another place. Being alone with your thoughts. My mind was at its most clear, I was relaxed, able to manage almost any thought that came into my head. Feeling my feet hit the pavement in a rhythm that was impossible to break, feeling my heart beat, feeling the wind or the sun hit my face or my back at a consistent pulse . . . it was serenity. It was . . . meditation.

I needed to lose weight and change my lifestyle— and fast. The next day, I joined a gym and signed up with a personal trainer.

After my twenty-eight days, I came home to New York City. By then, I had moved out of the home I shared with my wife and two boys and into a place of my own. And I stopped running completely. Like so many people who spend time in rehab, I relapsed (again, another story for another book). Thankfully, it was quick. After about three weeks of heavy drinking, I detoxed myself one night, woke up the next morning, and attended my first AA meeting outside of rehab. I was determined to stay sober this time. I had lost my job and my family and I was going to die if I relapsed again. To do this, all I had to do was one thing . . . go to a second meeting.

I did. At my second meeting in two days, I made a friend who soon became my sponsor. I shared how uneasy and anxious I felt, and the physical discomfort I was in (detoxing from alcohol without medication is difficult, but I chose that path as a deterrent for a future slip). His response was straightforward: "First, eat sugary foods like honey and chocolate (the physical detox from alcohol is actually from sugar not alcohol). Second, meditate." The sugary food was a simple fix (easiest advice I ever got), but the meditation would be hard, so that meant one thing: back to the treadmill. That was the beginning of the new me.

It became therapy for me. It was my release. It wasn't just the physical endorphin rush, but the feeling of accomplishment I'd have after the run.

Soon, I hit ninety meetings in ninety days, started working again, and was running every day. It wasn't much—three miles a day at a ten-minute pace, and always on the treadmill (running in New York City was nothing compared to running on the beach in Malibu). That all changed one fall day. A friend and I decided that we'd go on a run together, so we went to Central Park. I'd never even seen the running paths in Central Park, or what is more widely known as The Loop. Its 6.2 miles of relatively easy terrain, sans one quarter-mile stretch known as Cat Hill. That day, I didn't run the full loop (there are ways to shortcut the track and make it an even 5-mile run), but I couldn't believe it when I finished. First, it was the longest run I'd ever done. It took a little less than an hour but felt like twenty minutes. I had my music on, but no idea what songs I heard. There was nothing like it. That run changed me as a runner forever.

In Malibu, it was a straight shot—one mile out, one mile back, done. This was a labyrinth of different landscapes, statues, curves, and turns. It had inclines and declines. Running on a treadmill was exercise, running in Malibu was enlightening, running in Central Park was an experience. It also changed my mindset. Running outside in New York City is not the easiest, especially during the workweek, and though it's physically harder than the treadmill, to me it suddenly felt easier. I didn't realize it at the time, but running outside had become therapy, relaxation, it was my release. I began to savor my weekend runs, moving from the 5-mile shortcut to the full loop to what I call the corkscrew, which is the full 6.2-mile loop and a lap around the Jacqueline Onassis Reservoir in the middle of the park for another 1.6 miles. Add a little cutback and you get to 8 miles. Over time, running became "my time." As I was putting the pieces of my life back into place, focusing on my new job, putting my family back together and rebuilding friendships, running became my salvation. They say when you're an addict, you immediately feel your "fix" the minute you hear the sound of the bottle opening, before you even take the first sip. Running gave me that same feeling. Eventually, our

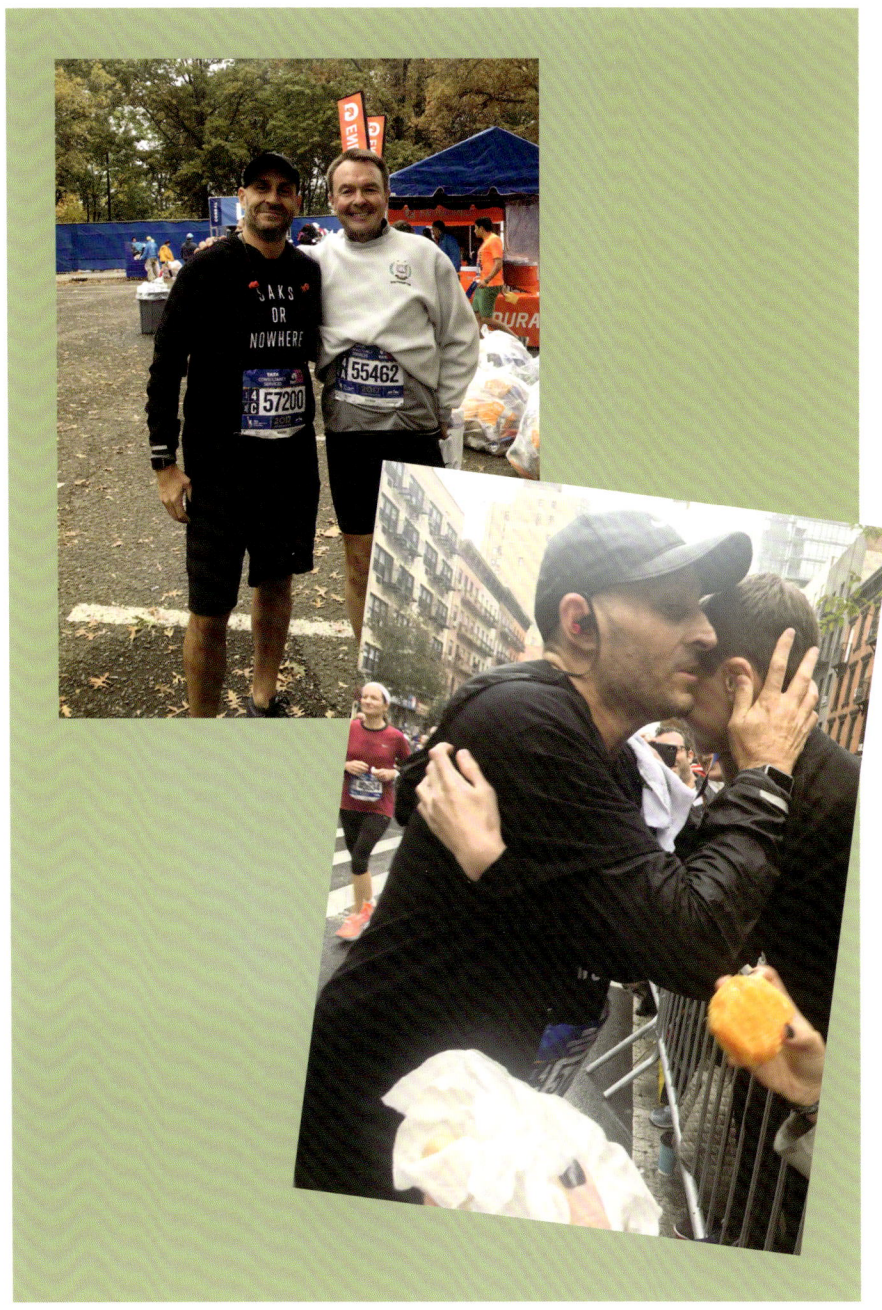

offices moved downtown, enabling me to run outside, along the Hudson River every day. First thing in the morning, in the rain, sleet, snow, or freezing cold, I relished those long runs outside during the week. They set me up for whatever the day ahead would bring. The mileage was increasing and that meant one thing: time to set a goal. I was going to run the NYC Marathon.

People say there's no feeling like it, especially if you live in New York. I have to say there was nothing like training for it. I loved the training regimen. The rigidity. The challenge every day. Unlike my normal routine, the training was different every day: some days were hills, some days were speed, some days were off, and some were long distance. With each week, there was more progress, longer runs, better times. After each run, I felt euphoric. I was getting the same high I'd get from drinking, but this was about wellness, achievement. It was good. An added benefit was what I got to see. Work takes me all over the United States and Europe. In the past when I was traveling, I'd stay in the hotel and run in the gym. With the marathon, I found myself needing longer runs during the week. I would run outside everywhere. I used to think there was no better feeling than running in Central Park. That was until I ran through Washington DC, from monument to monument, around the reflecting pool and down Pennsylvania Avenue. Running through Milan, Paris, Rome, Toronto, Berlin. Always alone, always at dawn. To me, there's no more of a serene feeling than running through Milan to the Duomo di Milano. I travel to Milan twice a year for business but never see any of the sights. On that morning, with peace and quiet, I spent a few minutes in the middle of my run just standing in the Piazza del Duomo. There was nothing like it.

The NYC Marathon was my most amazing run. It's a humbling concept, joining a race you know you have no chance of winning. I loved every minute of it. While I was training, all I would think about was what it would feel like to finish. But during the marathon, I savored the moment. It was clear I wasn't running to win, but unlike many others in the race, I wasn't running for a time goal, either. I was just running. Everyone who has run it has a different memory, a particular instance when they felt the power of the moment. As a New Yorker, I had a few eligible ones. For starters, I'd never been to Staten Island, or run across the Fifty-Ninth Street Bridge to 60,000 screaming fans cheering for me. But neither of those are my memory. For me, it was my wife, children, friends, and coworkers rooting me on at mile 17. Most of them have been with me, or at least knew me, when I was 320 pounds and an alcoholic—a walking warning sign. When I pulled over to the side to greet them, I could see it in their eyes. As I hugged my son, I pulled him close to me and said, "You can do anything you set your mind to, no matter what." That moment carried me the rest of the way, up First Avenue and through The Wall in the Bronx. I finished in 4:28:51. By far my slowest pace, about 15 minutes slower than my 20-mile training run. As I crossed the finish line, music off since mile 23, I could hear the roar of the crowd, all of it euphoric, all of it as I imagined.

The one feeling I didn't see coming was, "Now what?" Any runner knows what that means. That question is why very few people only run one marathon. I trained harder for the next one, this time for speed. I finished faster but missed my goal. You know what that means, right?

This was sort of a windy story, and I'm sorry, I'm not a writer. But I wrote this on an airplane flying back from a business trip to Paris. Just this morning, at 6 a.m., I ran down the Avenue George V, over the Pont de l'Alma to the left bank, down and around the Eiffel Tower, back up the left bank, up and over the Seine by way of Pont des Arts into the courtyard of the Louvre, out through the Jardin des Tuileries and back to my hotel. All I can say about that run is that I knew what I was going to write as my feet hit the ground for the first step into my run; it was like hearing the bottle open, even after all that time, both marathons, 110 pounds of weight loss, 4,169 miles logged, and 2,739 days of sobriety.

Marc Metrick, *forty-five, is the president of Saks Fifth Avenue. He resides on the Upper West Side of New York City with his wife, Deborah, and sons, Harrison, fifteen, and Charlie, ten.*

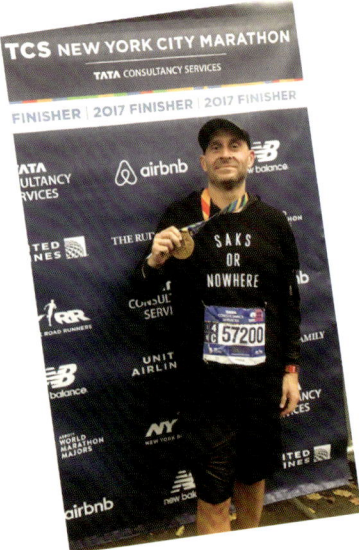

You Could Meet the Love of Your Life

George A. Hirsch

As spring 1988 approached, I and many other New-York-area running fans, began looking forward to the 1988 US Olympic Marathon Trials. The competition was scheduled to take place in April, with a beginning and end at Liberty State Park in New Jersey, just across the Hudson from Manhattan. That meant we could easily gain spectator access to what many believe to be the most exciting race in America.

Some of my friends planned to run the open marathon, but I hadn't gone the distance in four years nor trained for it, so I gave no thought to entering. I was psyched about the Trials marathon.

As the April date edged closer, our anticipation grew. Since I would be doing commentary for NBC at that summer's Olympic Games in Seoul, the Trials represented an important research opportunity for me. I had homework to do in New Jersey. It was a time for focus, attention, and analysis.

I didn't think for a moment about love. But life is so spectacularly unpredictable.

The day before the Sunday morning race, I joined several of my *Runner's World* colleagues at our booth in the race expo area at The Meadowlands. We were selling books and magazines, but mainly enjoying the chance to make new acquaintances and renew old friendships. Every Trials marathon brings out the most faithful—the runners and spectators who care deeply about US running and the Olympic Games.

I'm one of those. I had attended my first Olympic Games in Helsinki in 1952 and have been to many since. My life is filled with other interests and activities, but few make me happier than attending an Olympic Trials or Olympic Games.

I think you get the picture. I enjoyed greeting every passerby at the *Runner's World* booth. When Frank Shorter showed up, we fell into an elaborate discussion about the next day's marathon strategies. Who might go out fast and hard? Who would hang back early to save himself for a late charge? How would the American runners fare against their worldwide rivals in Seoul?

Frank and I have done this sort of analysis so often that it's like talking about the weather forecast. We ended our conversation by setting a dinner date for that evening.

I felt equally as engaged when chatting with a *Runner's World* subscriber I had just met for the first time. I was deep in conversation with one when, out of the corner of my eye, I spotted a dark-haired woman who paused at the booth. I had never seen her before but was immediately struck by her beauty, especially her radiant blue eyes.

We looked at each other briefly—and I know how this sounds; it sounds way too much like a cheesy Hollywood moment—but there was an instant connection between us. It was palpable. Then she continued her stroll through the expo. And all this while, I was still talking with the magazine subscriber.

Start slowly. Run a minute. Walk a minute.
Do that five times, then ten times, and reduce your
walking breaks. Keep a running diary.

As soon as that conversation ended, I hurried down the crowded expo aisles, looking for the radiant woman. After a few twists and turns, I spotted her and made a beeline to her side. "Hello," I said.

She was briefly startled, but then returned my greeting, and asked, "Are you George Hirsch?" Even if I hadn't been, I would have answered in the affirmative. I was just hoping for an opening that might lead to something more.

Lucky for me, she got things rolling. It turned out we had a mutual friend, and several months earlier that friend had asked me to supply a training plan for a first-time marathoner—the very woman I was face to face with now. Her name was Shay, and she simply wanted to thank me for sending along the marathon plan. She had followed it to a T, she told me, and was looking forward to testing its merits in the next morning's marathon.

"What's your goal time?" I asked, relieved to have such a simple conversation subject. Like all marathon novices, she answered, "I'm just hoping to feel good and go the distance." She hesitated for a moment, and then continued the thought: "If things go well, maybe I can run New York City in the fall, and try to qualify for Boston."

I should have responded with a few encouraging words, but the only thing that came out of my mouth was: "Would you like to have dinner tonight?" (Yes, I had already made plans with Frank Shorter, but we've been friends long enough that I knew he'd understand.)

Shay said no, she had to get home for the evening. I was disappointed but didn't give up, offering to walk her through a drizzle to her car in one of the mammoth parking lots. When we reached the car, wet and chilled, I asked if she would drive me back to the expo. I wasn't that concerned about the rain; I just wanted a few more minutes with her.

The next morning, I pulled on a T-shirt, sweatpants, and my training shoes and went looking for Shay at the start line. The weekend had begun as an Olympic scouting mission. Now I had something entirely different on my mind.

I watched the several hundred Trials racers take off, and then turned my attention to the open marathon with its three thousand participants, which started fifteen minutes later. I scanned the throng several times for Shay, but that proved futile. There were simply too many runners dressed in too many different kinds and colors of clothing.

That left me only one alternative: I walked to the back of the crowd and, after the starter's gun, I jogged across the line behind everyone else. Last place, that was me.

I was reasonably fit, thank goodness, and figured I would run at a slow steady pace until I caught up with Shay . . . somewhere along the course.

As I ran down the middle of the road, I spent so much time looking left and right that I worried my neck muscles might start cramping before my legs. But I was rewarded for my effort. After about five miles, I spotted Shay. She was running solo, deeply absorbed in her tunes, and seemed to be moving along smoothly.

Until I sauntered up beside her. "Hi. How you feeling?" I asked as nonchalantly as I could.

She was startled, needless to say. It took her a moment to find a response. Then she blurted out, "What are you doing here?"

"Well, to be honest, I'm looking for you," I said.

If you're just starting to run, the first thing is to get a good pair of shoes. Spend time at a running specialty store to get some good advice.

My candor might have scared her off, but fortunately didn't. It was a damp, windy day, and she was probably happy for the company. We fell into step, side by side, and began telling each other our life stories. The next fifteen miles flew by faster than any other run I had ever taken.

Just past the twenty-mile marker, the point of the infamous Wall, she said, "I'm getting tired."

I'm not sure what she wanted from me at that moment. Maybe some cheerleading. Maybe she wanted me to say, "Only six to go. You can do it." Or: "It's all downhill from here."

But for some reason, that's not what came to mind. While I definitely wanted to help Shay finish her marathon, the words that tumbled out were: "You're supposed to get tired. This is a marathon."

In retrospect, I'm lucky Shay ever spoke to me again. I remember that our chatter closed down the last six miles, as she turned inward to summon the grit she needed. We slowed a little but kept chugging onward. Eventually we saw the finish-line banner just ahead in a grassy field.

Since I wasn't wearing a race number, I stepped aside before the finish and melted into the spectators. Shay disappeared, too, but into the crowd of happy marathon runners who had successfully completed their day's business.

I held onto my last view of her. As she passed under the timing clock, it read 3:37:01—a Boston qualifying time. Then she was gone.

The next morning, it took me twice as long as usual to hobble the fifteen blocks to my office in midtown Manhattan. I was headed for a second cup of coffee when my phone rang. It was Shay. She was calling, she said, to thank me for helping her through the marathon.

The rest, as they say, is history. The following year, Shay Scrivner and I got married at The Boathouse in Central Park. That morning, several dozen friends had joined us for an "I ran with Shay and George on their wedding day" jog in the park. And we all have T-shirts to prove it.

I have run more than forty marathons in my life, in more than a half-dozen countries. But whenever someone asks me to name the most memorable, I don't have to think about it at all. I always answer, "That's an easy one."

George A. Hirsch, *chairman of the New York Road Runners, is a founder of the New York City five-borough marathon in 1976. He has run forty marathons with a personal best of 2:38 in Boston at age forty-four. Hirsch is the founding publisher of* New York *magazine, the long-time worldwide publisher of* Runner's World, *and was the first publishing director of* Men's Health *magazine.*

Running Exposed

Kelly McLay

I graduated from a reputable college youthfully invincible, knowing great things were in store. And they were; only the path to greatness was entirely unexpected. The next few years were defined by chaos physically and emotionally, and I was not prepared. For two years, this intense rollercoaster churned undiagnosed. I had no idea what was going on. My behavior was erratic and irrational. I was happy. I was sad. I was tired. I was snappy. I was surging hot only to become soaking wet and freezing cold. I constantly tried to ground myself, but the world kept spinning. I felt crazy. I am, a little bit, but this was out-of-control crazy. My friends and family would define these times as my "hot mess" years, and rightly so. It wasn't pretty. I wasn't bleeding profusely from a gaping wound, but this was not me. After a year of gaining almost forty-five pounds, hibernating daily, and finally seeking a second opinion from a physician who would listen, I received the diagnosis.

I had gone through menopause.

I was twenty-four.

Your twenties are meant to be a little crazy, right? Filled with newfound income, city life, parties, sex, alcohol . . .not night sweats, mammograms, and kegel balls. Friends were out partying, avoiding pregnancy at all costs, and I was desperately trying to hold onto any last flicker of fertility. My mind couldn't digest the full magnitude nor was my body capable of coping. I neither fit in with the twenty-year-old hysterectomy cancer patients nor the fifty-five-year-old menopausal likes of my mom and her friends. Okay, I did attend the play "Menopause" with them at twenty-five, and it was the most awkward and amazing night for me with this group of women who carried me under their hot, sometimes sweaty, wings. But laughs aside, a part of me had died. My womanhood, my female privilege, my future dreams, my physical youthfulness . . . gone. I had always wanted kids, several, and that was gone. My heart broke and so did my body. Guilt consumed my heartache, because this wasn't a death sentence, but trying to rise above the physical and emotional scars to control this imbalance felt hopeless.

That year, and many years to follow, were filled with confusion. And wine. A lot of wine. Maybe too much wine. The spontaneous, athletic, social, outgoing, fun-

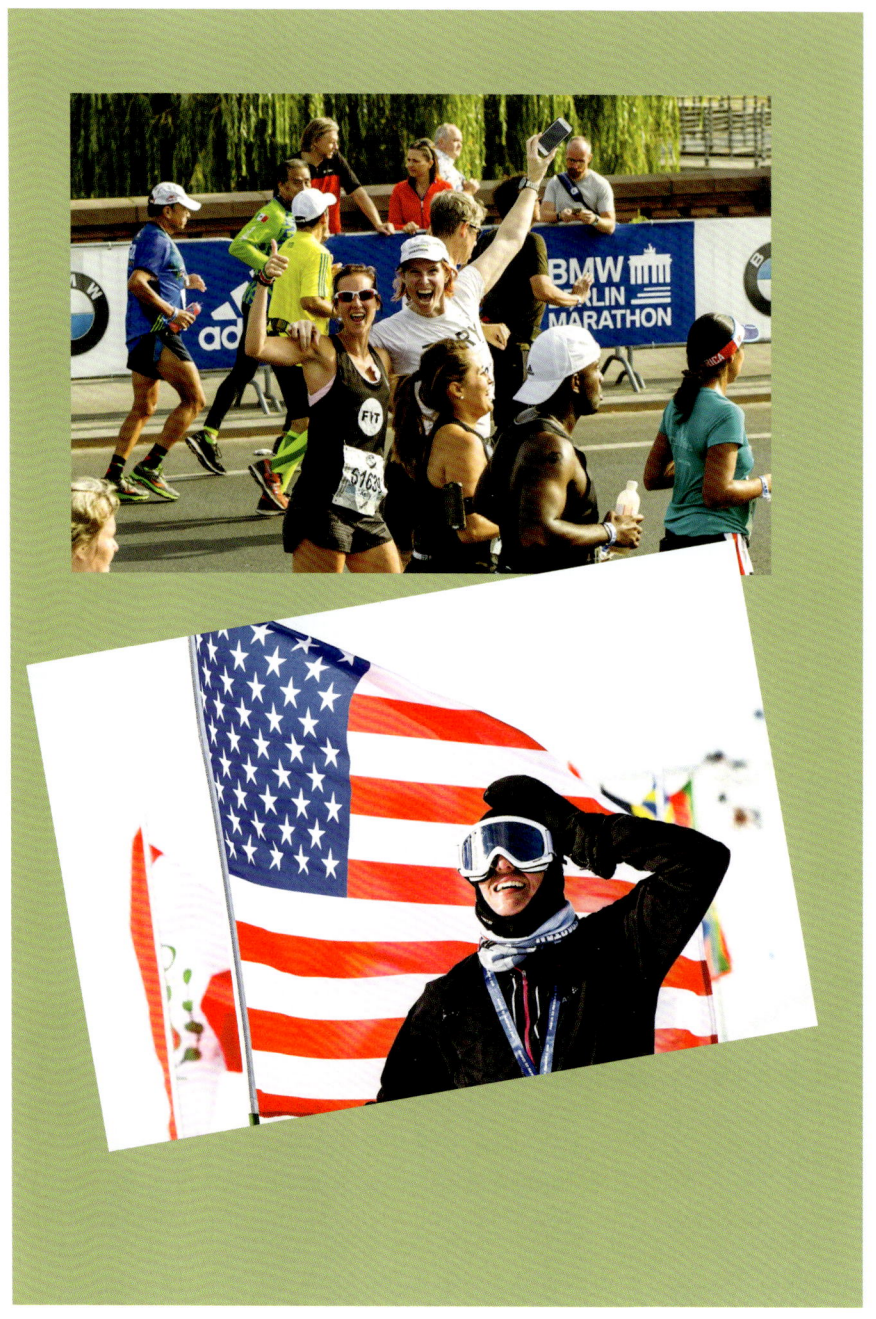

loving, multitasking Kelly was unrecognizable. My life was spiraling and I needed a goal. Insert: the Marathon. Big Goal.

I latched onto my sisters' group of friends, who were training for the Boston Marathon at the time. For someone who was an athlete all her life, I was desperately out of shape. Having said that, I didn't run. In high school, I joined the track team and lasted all of two weeks. That first mile was painful. I didn't make it. I felt like crawling. My lungs burned and my legs stung. I hated every minute of running. If three miles felt unattainable, the marathon . . . well, that was just dumb. I felt defeated, in so many ways, but I needed the pain. And so, I ran.

Save the running selfie. See the world. See things with your own eyes. Take one picture, then put the phone away. Document a run with your soul.

I ran far. In the cold, in the rain, in the heat, five miles, ten miles, twenty miles . . . as far as I could go. Each longer mile introduced a new pain, and each breakthrough a new challenge conquered. There's something very beautiful about running the snowy silence of winter, facing your greatest challenges head on. I ran through failure. I ran through defeat. I ran through tears and insignificance, heartache and embarrassment. I had left college with such invincibility and here I was falling apart—no job, a few friendships on the brink, no confidence. I pounded the pavement as hard as I could. To escape. To expunge. There was a lot of healing in those solitary miles. The repetition of each foot strike against the pavement healed a bit of me with each step. And step by step that pain got me to the very famous "right on Hereford, left on Boylston." When I turned that corner and the blue and yellow arches hovered in the near distance, my throat choked up and I burst into tears. The ugliest crying and most beautiful tears one could ever know. The weight of the past two years lifted off my shoulders as the finish time clicked. A finish line that seemed so impossible. Running opened the door to possible.

Running became such a natural part of my day, a moment I most looked forward to. The movement of my body against the hard grain felt amazing. Alone on the roads, I had the freedom to explore more of myself and more of the environment around me. I could push myself when I needed to cut through the pain, or I could choose to float on the cadence of each step. I reached such natural highs and felt empowered. There was a difference now: I wanted to run. I wanted the pain for its return of accomplishment. Running gave back what I was willing to put in. It inspired me to own the diagnosis; to allow it to empower a definition of who I was and where I was going. And I owned it.

I shared it freely and openly and, as such, the very first weekend I met my husband, he knew exactly what he was getting into.

By now, I absolutely loved running. I valued the heartache that got me there, as that very passion led me straight into a career of running and travel. It was surreal; my friends were in disbelief. How did I manage to turn my passion into my profession? Soon, one marathon turned into twenty, which turned into forty, which over time organically earned me five world majors and six continents and a camaraderie of runners larger than I could ever imagine. This magic of running morphed into a shared endeavor. I found I could share this passion with others as we traveled the world fully immersed in the culture around us. Running broke down any barriers, allowing us to interact in such a human way. The happiness of Kenya, the dreams of Australia, the respect of Japan, the spontaneity of Chile, the history of Europe, each challenging our own cultures in such amazing ways. Seeing the sun beam off Fuji, getting kissed by the island winds of exotic Rapa Nui, and set in the grasslands of Africa as you watch the gentle breathing of a female pride. Us runners, on this journey together, were so lucky. We shared such intimate experiences, ending days fascinated by what we saw and who we met, pinching ourselves for this life over laughter and wine. And running opened this world. It's a beautiful thing seeing the world by foot.

Run naked. There is a time and place for gadgets, but 95 percent of my runs are tech free. Footprint the world.

Work and running were one in the same. Every waking moment was dedicated to living and breathing these two; I loved showing people the world, I loved celebrating their accomplishments, and I enjoyed meeting so many diverse people. It soon became very apparent to me that the more successful I was, the more I was exposed to criticism and manipulation in a work environment that became increasingly impossible. I wasn't smart enough, I wasn't strong enough, I wasn't capable, I was a woman, I wanted children . . .More than once, my confidence was shot down. The writing was on the wall after my first journey to Antarctica with a running tour company. I was offered a once in a lifetime opportunity not only to travel to Antarctica, but to run a marathon there. I couldn't believe it. First, when in my life did I ever think I would travel to Antarctica, let alone have such an incredible goal so tangible?

The day before the race, like a kid on Christmas morning, I inquired as to what day was best for me to partake? The response was short. The race was for the clients, not me. I just stood there, dumbfounded. I kept a brave face on each day during the marathon, celebrating with clients as they reached their finish line. Completing a marathon on all seven continents was never originally a goal—it just happened organically, turning into an unbelievable goal. When I learned from my company's management that I would not be able to complete all 7 continents by running Antarctica, it cut me to the core. I had no idea if I would ever make it back—the bottom of the world is neither the easiest nor most affordable of destinations—but that moment made it very clear I had to leave this new job. Running was again at the forefront of coping. Finding some way to stay strong, find a voice, and have the courage to leave something I absolutely loved. So, I left; one race short of seven continents, one race shy of the world marathon majors, and one baby short of our family. I sobbed every step of the way. I was so lucky and I was so blessed. But I wanted more, I needed more . . . and I deserved more.

As far as you run, you cannot outrun reality. And the reality was that there remained a few goals: seven continents and motherhood. The journey to motherhood is impossible to prepare for in the most straightforward of situations. Embarking on this path meant facing menopause head on. That's when unsolicited commentary on my running through infertility started happening. From nurses questioning why I would risk everything, to one woman recommending I should just stop running and eat a burger. Mmmm . . . is that all? That would be amazing. I'd eat all the burgers in the world if that was the trick! So many assumed my infertility resulted from my marathoning. How far from the truth. But truly, stop running? My whole means of survival from the loss I felt was running.

If the menopause rollercoaster prepared me for anything, it was the ups and downs of infertility, specifically IVF via donor egg. Running gave me the optimism that everything would work out, and I carried that strength through every obstacle over the next two years: through the legal papers, the loans, the tests and more tests; when the finances required cash, when the lawyers said not to trust the donor, when the pain of the needles dug deep into my nerves, running powered me on. When it was finally our turn and our donor was ready for surgery, and all the eggs, her eggs, were destroyed. We had finally made it to the day, and the retrieval epically failed. When we thought it was over, she committed to trying again. Five days after the transfer, I ran a half-marathon with my best friend and told her it worked. And it did. Despite outside scrutiny and with the support of my immediate physician group and husband, I continued running through my pregnancy. It wasn't until twenty-seven weeks after I crossed the finish line of the 2016 Dublin Marathon that we announced our pregnancy. I guess until that finish line, we didn't think it was really happening.

Then I received a chance call one day from a race director looking for someone experienced in global marathons to assist with his company. I was ecstatic. The bonus—a trip to Antarctica to understand his event and allow me to finish my seventh continent. Oh my . . . sweet karma. So that's why, years later, standing at the bottom of the world in sub-zero temperatures, I broke down and cried. I had no idea how I was ever going to finish. But I did, I made it taking one step forward each day.

After Antarctica, I went on to even greater achievements, finishing seven marathons on seven continents in seven days, becoming one of twenty-five women in the world who can claim the honor. I couldn't believe I did it! More importantly, I did this just thirteen months after having my daughter. A month after this huge personal accomplishment and spending too long removed from the industry I so very loved, I launched F.I.T. (Fitness International Travel) bringing runners, friends, and family to global marathons, and I haven't looked back.

It wasn't that long ago women were battling for the opportunity to run. It's pretty incredible how far we have come, and yet I find some days I am battling the similar obstacles. But I am proud to be part of this force. I hope I am continuing to carry the running torch to open the doors for women—athletes, executives, moms. And while I have some very supportive men around me, some I am forever indebted to, it has been the women around me that have resurrected my strength. Have you ever watched a pack of runners stride in unison? When I was running in Kenya, the lead males passed me with such graceful power, gaining energy from one another as they paced into the distant sunrise. It was mesmerizing. It's easy to feed off the power of running in a group, each of you beating in sync as you move together toward a collective goal. I have hugged strangers at the end of a race who strode every 26.2 with me. That's the thing about running, its language is innate to us as humans. It has no barriers; it is multi-lingual, it is fluid, it is malleable. Running evens the playing field. It is accessible—tall or small, young or old, rich or poor—we can all touch it.

Back to that day in Antarctica: I was exposed. To the elements. To the root of what running is to me. All that I was told was impossible found possibility at finish line after finish line. I realized then, all that time I wasn't running away from anything, I was running to something greater. I learned so much about myself, my strength, community, and life—the running was to endure. I was exposed to greatness, to my body feeling as strong as it could possibly be. Running has shown me a world of opportunity.

Running means the world to me; it is both my heartbeat and my breath. The pain, the freedom, the high, the raw nature of it removing layers until your core is both exposed and empowered. Running has taught me a lot about pain and perseverance. Running is raw, not allowing you to hide from reality while physically empowering you to cope with its presence. At peak exertion you find sheer bliss, like the eye of a tornado, clarity. In that moment of seeming defeat surges great resilience. The moment is foggy. Until you find a way to break through, where purpose and confidence await at the finish. This raw exposure is what makes it real, makes me real. This is the running I savor. These moments offer clarity and confidence that inspire me to leap.

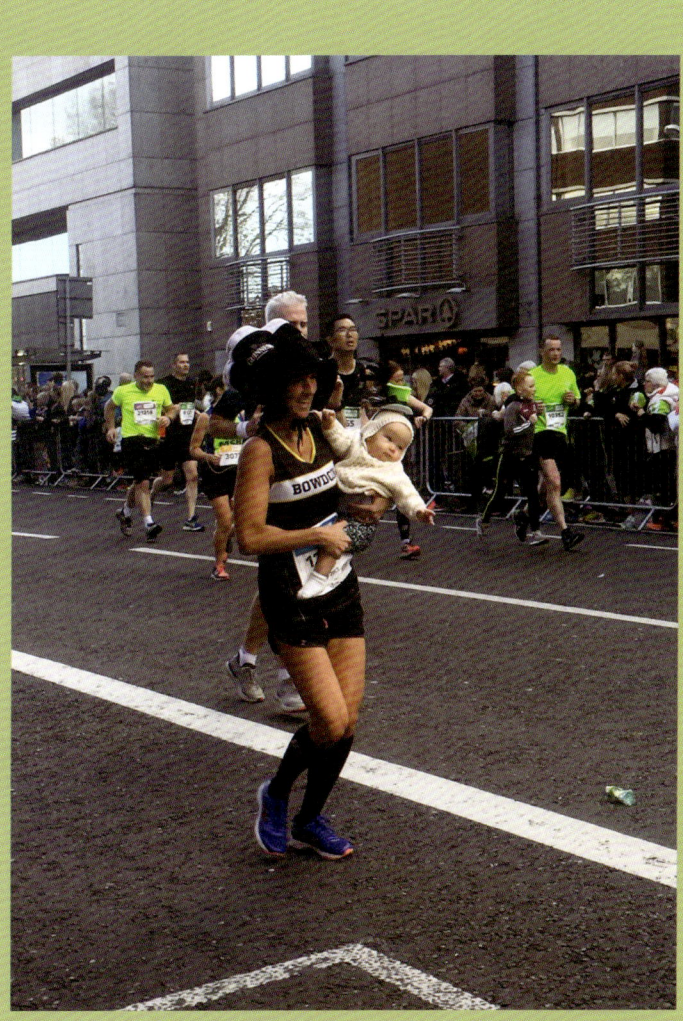

Run your life, don't let others run you.

Life will always have its obstacles. Despite beating the impossible these past few years—motherhood, Antarctica, the World Marathon Challenge—there is still more to conquer. The barriers I am facing seem insurmountable—career setbacks, multiple miscarriages, challenging corporate politics for the female entrepreneur—and so I continue to lace up because it makes me happy and it makes others happy, and that is the key to life. I am the best, strongest, and most capable version of me when I run. If I run, I can do anything.

I am proud to be this woman.

I am proud of all my mistakes and all my ugly moments.

I am proud of the run that got me here.

On October 29, 2017, thirteen years and two days to the day I found out about menopause, I crossed the finish line of the Dublin Marathon holding my baby girl in my arms and carrying my favorite title: Mom. It was absolutely beautiful and the proudest moment of my life. My journey had truly come full circle.

Kelly McLay *is the founder of Fitness International Travel and passionate about the marathon distance. With sixty-five-plus marathon completions, Kelly is a two-time seven-continent marathoner and one of only forty women in the world to complete the World Marathon Challenge: seven marathons on seven continents in seven days. Kelly is a graduate of Bowdoin College and resides just north of Boston with her husband, John, and baby, Scarlett.*

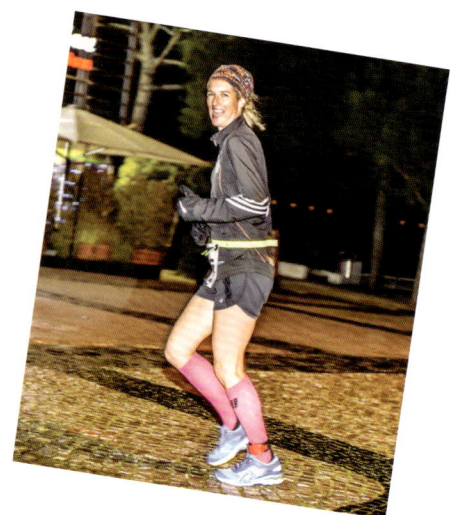

Life Is Full of Choices: I Chose to Run

Michael Rodgers

My running story is my life story. When I was younger, I didn't openly share much about my background and why I started running. I realized, as time passed, that when I did recount the "how I started and why I run," it helped me, and in turn it helped others, too. I would get varied reactions: some were impressed by my accomplishments, others just seemed to enjoy my running versions of "fishing tales," but then there were others . . . the people that seemed to see themselves, who connected to the "why" in my reason for running. People in this latter group would often open up and share their running/life stories. My hope in sharing my story is that it will serve as an inspiration to others to find their passion and happiness, hopefully in running.

Let's go back to the beginning, 1975. My mother graduated from high school in June, but she wasn't headed to college. I was born two months later. She was eighteen years old, with a newborn child. She had a lot to figure out in order to take care of and provide for me.

> *My hope in sharing my story is that it will serve*
> *as an inspiration to others to find their passion and*
> *happiness, hopefully in running.*

Obvious curiosity probably leads you to the question, what about my father? Well, this is the part of my story that I buried in a pile of shame for years. It's not that I didn't know who he was; rather, he wasn't present—at all. Growing up, I would hear great stories about my dad and how much of an amazing athlete he was. I would go to my grandparents' house and see his memorabilia and trophies, but it was just metal and plastic. My father was just a picture on the wall, the script on an award nameplate. He was only there one time, and that visit was filled with many awkward, silent moments.

I made multiple attempts to start a relationship with him, but to no avail. I only got to know my father through secondhand stories. While most of them were about his stellar athletic prowess, eventually they transitioned to how sad it was that he wasted his talent. My dad was hailed as the best all-around athlete from his town, region, and even state. It turned out that none of these things would have an impact on him as the defining moment in his life, when his mother passed away. He was devastated, and while many of his other friends were going to parties and making normal, young partygoer mistakes, he took it to the next level. This lifestyle quickly led to drug and alcohol addiction. Prison followed for a period of time, and the choices he made in life, whether directly or indirectly related to his battle with addiction, made it such that I was never going to develop a relationship with him.

He was devastated, and while many of his other friends were going to parties and making normal, young partygoer mistakes, he took it to the next level.

As a kid, that was tough. I would see kids doing things with their fathers. Granted, my mother did get married and had my two brothers; however, my stepfather and I never developed a strong bond, and I never viewed him as "my" father. My mother ended up divorced from my stepfather, and once again was a single mother, but this time of three boys. She reverted to "figure it out" mode.

She provided for us, working long hours at her full-time job and occasional part-time jobs, too. As the oldest, I was often responsible for cooking for my brothers, helping with homework, leading the effort to get household chores done, etc. I'll admit, I wasn't always the nicest of big brothers. There were times when I would torment my brothers, saying the dishes weren't clean, making them rewash them just for the heck of it. Mean, I know, but that's what big brothers do, right? It wasn't the most ideal childhood, but it wasn't the worst either.

I was a decent student; however, I struggled with a learning disability. I was always a grade level or two behind in reading and was the student who got pulled out of class for special education help. My worst nightmare came to life when the teacher would go around the class, making everyone read a paragraph. I would stumble over words and my classmates would make fun of me. I used to count ahead to see what paragraph I would have to read so I could practice. Sometimes it worked, too often it didn't.

Now that you have a bit of backstory on my childhood, let's get to the point where running entered my life. Throughout elementary school, I did look forward to the President's Physical Fitness mile in gym class. That was the day I exceled, no reading ahead, stumbling, or shame. I was always one of the fastest kids, and some years *the* fastest. Our annual spring field day was my favorite day of the year. That was the day I got to run races and win ribbons—the most cherished of which was that blue first-place ribbon—and be noticed for something other than the kid with a learning disability. Sometimes, I would settle for a red second-place ribbon, but the best was riding the school bus home with multiple blue ribbons. I longed for field day every year, the day other kids didn't make fun of me.

Fast forward to sixth grade, age eleven. I took home a piece of paper about running indoor track. I had played soccer for many years, but running was what I loved. I begged my mom to sign me up for the team. She did with one stipulation: I had to get good grades. If I didn't study hard, do my homework, and pay attention in school, I couldn't run. That's all I needed to hear. I vowed to put my nose to the grind and study hard.

I went from a kid who struggled in school with special ed classes to an honors student-athlete. By the time I was a senior in high school, I was the four-time MVP of my cross-country team, an 800m state finalist on the track, and voted by my peers as the male athlete of the year. More importantly, my course load was packed with AP or honors classes.

Running provided me the opportunity to thrive, on the track and in the classroom. It was something I was good at and I got a lot of attention, exactly what every teenager wants. I will forever be grateful to my mother for dangling the carrot of running in front of my face and forcing me to focus on my studies and education.

In middle and high school, I ran with the same group of guys. We were friends but not best friends. Our friendship was all about running. We ran at cross-county or track practice after school. We would crack jokes and gossip on the runs, then go back to our respective friend groups. We had a healthy, friendly competition. Some meets I would be first on the team, others I would be second, just like those field days in elementary school. At the end of meet, we would all congratulate each other, say good race, and life went on.

Running provided me the opportunity to thrive, on the track and in the classroom.

Although I was a good runner, I wasn't the best of the best. I didn't get recruited to run at a Division I school. In fact, I only had one Division III school send me a letter about running. I was good enough to walk on to my college cross-country team. I would consistently run between two and four on the team. I did my part, but I wasn't having fun. Granted, I don't think any collegiate athlete likes waking up early to run workouts before class in addition to showing up in the afternoon for another workout. It was more than that: I'd lost that collegial sense of "we're here because we love to run and have fun." It wasn't enjoyable anymore. I'd became disillusioned with running. I stopped running on the team after my freshman year.

But I didn't stop running. I just stopped running on the team. I wasn't running races anymore; I just ran when I felt like it. I ran when I wanted to feel good. I ran for me, because I loved to run.

Jump to several years after college, and I'm still running occasionally when I need to get my fix of a runner's high. I visited a friend in Minnesota, whom I accompanied to watch one of her friends run Grandma's Marathon. We drove to Duluth the day before the race and stayed in a house with a group of people running the full and half marathon. That night over dinner, one of the guys in the house decided he wasn't running. He'd registered, but didn't train, so he offered up his bib to anyone who wanted to run the half. The longest run I'd ever done was an eleven-mile training run back in high school. Even though I was only running occasionally at the time, I decided "why not?"

> *I wasn't running races anymore; I just ran when I felt like it. I ran when I wanted to feel good. I ran for me, because I loved to run.*

Yes, this is a public confession that my first half marathon was run as a bandit under someone else's bib. At the time, I didn't realize the implications, and of course if I knew then what I know now, it never would have happened. I digress . . .

My first half marathon was a blast. I ran the early miles by myself, scared. Would I be able to make it to the finish? I soon started running and talking with a guy. We were two chatter boxes getting to know each other. At mile eight, he encouraged me to go ahead. I declined, saying it was still a way to go and I wanted to keep running with him. He also tried at mile nine to get me to go ahead, again, I refused. At mile ten, he made it clear that our time together was over. He started walking. I was on my own. Realizing there was only a 5k to go, I thought, "I can do that. It's just as long as a high school cross-country race." I took off! I was passing so many people along the way. I don't remember my splits, but I'm sure I negative spilt that race.

I was sore after the race, but I had a blast. Just over two years later, I ran the Niagara Falls Half Marathon and cut nine minutes off my time. Energized by my success, I was hooked, and thus began my road-running career.

By this time, I'd moved to New York City for my job. I remember bragging to one of my colleagues about my recent half marathon. She told me if I liked running, I had to

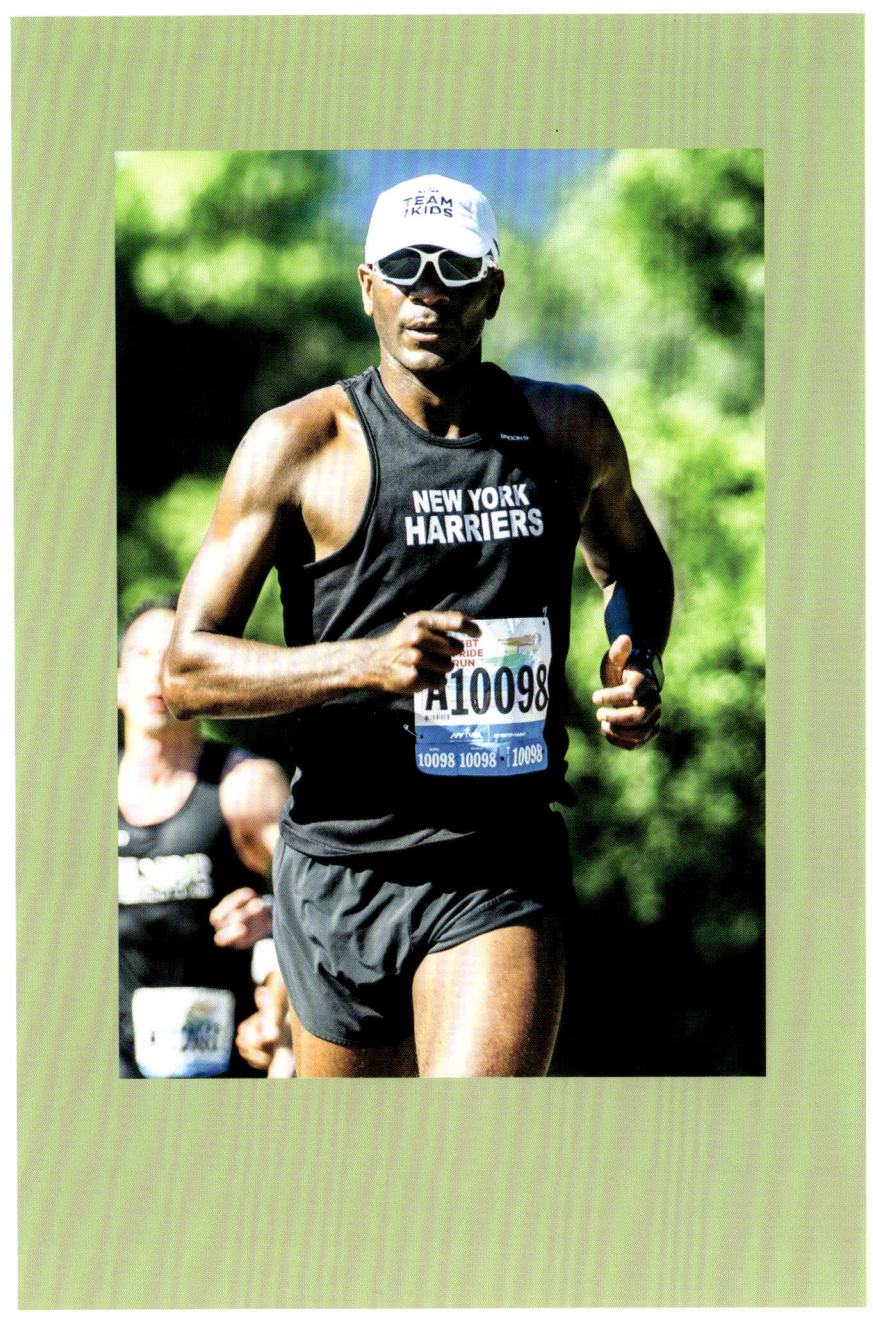

look up New York Road Runners (NYRR) because they put on races all the time. I soon learned NYRR was the organization that put on the New York City Marathon. I thought it could be fun to run some of their races, but not the marathon. Remember, I was an 800m guy. Granted, I was the one walking around work bragging about running a half marathon, but a full marathon, that would be crazy.

> *I took off! I was passing so many people along the way. I don't remember my splits, but I'm sure I negative spilt that race.*

On November 2, 2003, I was on the subway headed to The Cloisters with a friend visiting from Europe for a picnic lunch. We were headed north from my apartment in the Financial District and noticed it was much more crowded than usual. Unbeknownst to us, it was marathon Sunday. We changed our destination and went into Central Park to see the race. We ended up standing at mile twenty-four, cheering and high-fiving runners for hours. Fortunately, we had our picnic lunch and a bottle of wine. That was the day I changed my mind about marathons. I was mesmerized by the thousands of runners streaming by us. There were people of all shapes and sizes from around the world. Some runners were charging through the park, while others were walking one step at a time toward the finish line. I was in awe. I told myself, "I must do this!"

The next fall, I ran the Marine Corps Marathon. Six months later, the Paris Marathon. Six months after that, the Chicago Marathon. A year later, the New York City Marathon. I'd been bitten by the marathon bug. I had fallen in love with running again. It was fun to travel with my mother and run marathons all over, but even more fun training and preparing for the races. Running was again a focal point in my life. It was something I could do anywhere. While at home in New York City, or traveling around the country or world with my job as a nonprofit fundraising consultant. I loved it.

I joined NYRR to get the member discount for the weekly races in Central Park and around the city. I used the races as training runs and to check in on my progress toward my goal of running a Boston Marathon qualifying time, which I did at the Berlin Marathon in 2007. I'll never forget the tears of joy I cried when I saw my mother at mile 25.5 of that race. I hugged her and said, "We're going to Boston!"

I had trained for years by myself. Something I missed as part of running was the camaraderie of a team. As I was training for my first Boston Marathon, I joined the New York Harriers. Unlike my college team, the Harriers were the perfect mix of people who loved running, training hard, and having fun. The team trained three times a week but also had plenty of social events. My favorite of which was the monthly social, First Thursday, hosted by different members at their favorite bar in the city. This was the balance I needed. There were fast runners to challenge me and keep me grounded. I might be a Boston qualifier, but I was still getting my butt handed to me. Post-workout I would head to the bar for dinner and drinks with the same guys who just dusted me on the track.

I continued running marathons, twenty to date. Three memorable moments that stand out for me as a marathoner are qualifying for my first Boston, breaking the three-hour mark in Boston, and earning my Abbott World Marathon Majors Six-Star medal.

I had achieved my goals in marathoning and was open to a new challenge. I remember doing a long run with a group of guys from the Harriers and hearing one of them talk about his IRONMAN training. I had heard of an IRONMAN and knew it was a triathlon, but really didn't know the distances. When he told me the race was a 2.4-mile swim, a 112-mile bike, and a marathon (26.2 miles), I immediately responded, "That's stupid! Why would anyone ever do that?" Yes, that's the same question I used to ask about people who ran marathons. I'm pretty sure you already figured out that I would eventually set a goal of finishing an IRONMAN.

I didn't jump right in, because remember, I thought it was a stupid idea. It took a bit of time. My first triathlon was in 2010. My best friend convinced me to do a sprint tri. After that race, I thought to myself, "Okay, maybe a half-IRONMAN wouldn't be so bad." Three months later, I completed my first half-IRON distance race. Following that race, I signed up for a full IRONMAN in August 2011.

This was the balance I needed. There were fast runners to challenge me and keep me grounded.

I have an addictive personality; once I get the taste for something new and it's a challenge, I'm all over it. I have now completed five full IRONMAN races, including IRONMAN Boulder on my fortieth birthday. For that race, I raised money to support NYRR's youth programs. Thanks to the generosity of my friends and family, we raised over fifteen thousand dollars and adopted a school in Brooklyn that was part of the program. A few months later, I went to visit the school, and we gave each kid in the school a free pair of running shoes. This was by far one of my best birthdays ever.

Running had become more than a hobby; my lifestyle revolved around running. I was fortunate enough to land a job at New York Road Runners, where I'm able to combine my years of nonprofit fundraising experience and passion, some would say obsession, for running. I never would have imagined I'd find myself working in running, but I love it and am so grateful to go to work every day to help and inspire people through running, NYRR's mission.

There are many highlights to my job. I get to meet thousands of runners with incredible stories about why they run. I often stand at the finish lines of NYRR races, including the New York City Marathon, congratulating runners and greeting them with a high-five and/or hug. I believe every finish line is worth celebrating, whether it's a new PR or a race that didn't go as planned. The fact that you started and finished is an achievement. Through NYRR Team for Kids, the organization's charity running team, I get to help people train for races and watch them gain self-confidence through running, all while raising money to support youth running programs for kids like me years ago.

Running had become more than a hobby; my lifestyle revolved around running.

Probably the best part of my job is working with our various free youth and community programs. These programs include Run for the Future, a scholarship program for girls in their senior year of high school who are new to running; Open Run, a weekly community-based walk/runs in local parks; and Striders, the walking program for seniors. The largest is Rising New York Road Runners, which impacts hundreds of thousands of kids every year. There are a lot of running-based activities in the program; however, it's much broader than running. The program is designed to build kids' physical literacy, developing their skills, motivation, and desire to be physically active for life. Whether they become lifelong runners like me or not, hopefully they'll learn to enjoy moving and being active. The program is currently in more than 1,300 schools and community centers in 47 states, the District of Columbia, and Puerto Rico.

As part of my job, I visit sites using the program and have the opportunity to speak to students. Sometimes it's a school assembly, a graduation ceremony, or as part of a shoe giveaway; NYRR has given away over twenty thousand pairs of running shoes to kids in our programs. The message I share with the students is about choices. I share my story and use it as an example to emphasize to them that they always have a choice.

It's a simple message; however, when I share it in the context of my life/running story, it seems to resonate with people. By opening up about my past, of having a supportive mother encouraging me, while only hearing stories of an absent father, I become a real person not just another guest speaker. They pay attention and listen because they can relate. I'm someone like them. That's my opportunity to share my love of running and the importance of choices.

Because of running, I chose to study and became an honors student. I was the first person in my mother's family to graduate from college. I didn't go to school on a full-ride running scholarship, but as an honors fellow. Because of running, I chose not to drink alcohol at parties in high school. I chose to not smoke cigarettes or pot. I chose not to use steroids to get stronger and faster. These were all conscious decisions, ones I'm glad I made. Some of my peers, family and friends, made other choices. Because of their choices, many of them didn't excel in school and some even spent months to years in jail.

Don't get me wrong, my life isn't perfect. My father recently passed. I never did get to know him personally. That sucks and hurts. How did I deal with it? I chose to run. Some may say I was running from my feelings. On the contrary: for me, when I run, I feel. I feel the only connection to my father I know, our shared athleticism. I feel my self-esteem growing like it did when I would win those ribbons at field day. I feel my mother's pride as she watches me cross finish lines. I feel the dignity of knowing that by going to work every day and running for NYRR Team for Kids, I'm helping other kids find their happy, safe place away from bullying classmates or less than ideal home situations.

With all of the choices I've had in life, I chose to run. I am forever grateful for the focus, opportunities, and fun it has brought to my life. I hope that my story will influence others to make positive choices that help them find their passion, guiding them toward happiness. If it's running, like it was for me, I will gladly invite you on a run so we can share miles and stories.

Michael Rodgers *is an active member of the New York City running community. Rodgers serves as vice president of youth and community runner engagement at New York Road Runners. He manages a variety of programs that offer the running community opportunities to actively support NYRR's mission to help and inspire people through running. He has completed twenty-five marathons, five IRONMAN triathlons, and one ultra-marathon.*

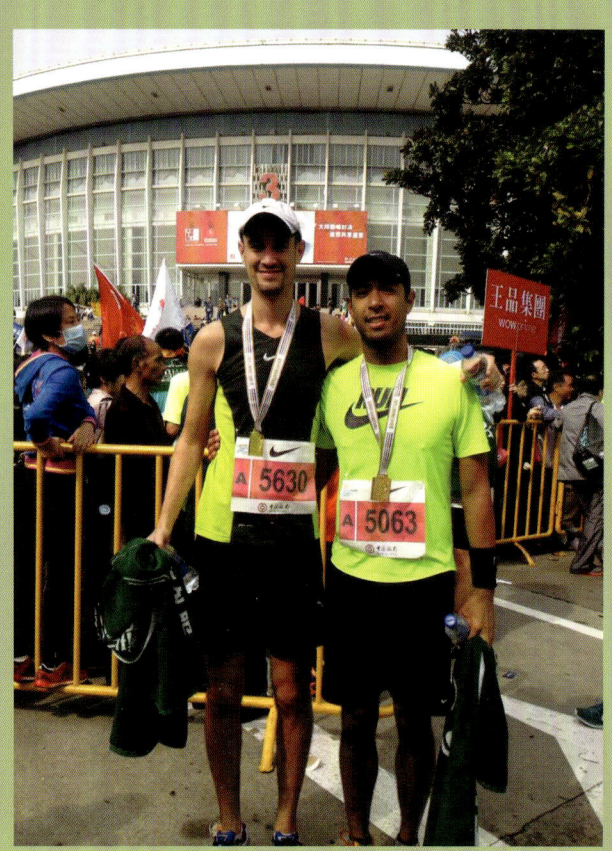

*But deep down inside, I was never comfortable,
and I did not know whether to face my fear of
who I really was or to continue running away.*

When the Finish Line Is Just the Beginning

Joe Suntharaphat

During my second year of college, I realized that I owned the decisions I made (especially regarding my health). Freshman year was the year of overconsumption, late-night study sessions which often involved food and unhealthy eating habits. It was not until after I left the dormitory that I was resolved to do something to change my habits and lifestyle. I saw running as an activity that would not only help me lose weight, but also achieve a healthy lifestyle.

To be honest, I never understood running. In high school, I had a few friends who were on the track and cross-country teams. I thought to myself, *Why would anyone want to run as a sport?* It seemed to be a fruitless and exhausting activity with no end goal. I was fortunate enough to attend a college with close proximity to beautiful hiking and running trails along the Pacific Coast. It served not only as motivation, but also seemed to be a good distraction from the actual act of running.

After a couple years of off-and-on running, I decided to push myself and enter a full marathon. I didn't know what I was getting myself into. I had loosely followed a training plan, but my ego assured me that running 26.2 miles would be easy. I didn't know about all the other ancillary preparation one's body needed to go through, both physical and mental.

I showed up on race day, and the energy at the start line was incredible. I was nervous, excited, and ready to go. I started a bit too fast, and at the halfway mark, my body started to show signs of wear. My legs started cramping, I was poorly hydrated, and I was chafing in places I thought I would never chafe. At mile fifteen, my legs seized. I fell to the ground and literally had to roll off to the side to avoid getting ran over. Passing runners were yelling at me to "walk it off!", but I was completely incapacitated.

After a few minutes of rolling around and resting my legs, I was able to get up and slowly walk off the pain. I crossed the finish line with blood on my shirt and dust all over my body and clothes; I looked like I had just come from a war zone. I was certain this would be my first and last marathon.

Because I enjoyed the solitary endeavor of running, it gave me plenty of time to think. I had already been running a marathon for most of my adult life. I had a feeling that I was gay during my junior high school years but did not know if the feelings were real or whether they would fade away. When I entered high school (an all-boys high school), I found my attraction to boys grow stronger but did my best to suppress those feelings.

I wanted to fit in with the rest of my friends and classmates. I played team sports and socialized with girls from our sister schools. But deep down inside, I was never comfortable, and I did not know whether to face my fear of who I really was or to continue running away.

> *But deep down inside, I was never comfortable, and I did not know whether to face my fear of who I really was or to continue running away.*

Having grown up in an Asian household, my focus was to study, obtain good grades, and attend college. I graduated from high school and thought I could start fresh in college. Regrettably, I felt more pressure to conform. I continued to fight my attraction to guys and focused again on my studies and hanging out with friends. It was not until I started running in college that I had time to focus on me. Often on my runs, I would imagine what my life would be like in the future. Focused on thinking about what I could change and how to deal with the change. I graduated college and still had not come out.

A few years later, I moved to Boston for graduate studies and that was a real test for me. I was in a new environment and did not know anyone on the East Coast. Perhaps I could finally be myself. It didn't happen right away. I continued to run and my attraction to men only grew stronger. I started working out, and that was when I had mustered enough courage to ask out a guy who had caught my eye at the gym. I was so nervous. What if he wasn't gay? What if he was dating someone already? What if . . .? We met up for dinner and drinks, and we had a great time. It was such a relief to finally be able to be with someone to whom I could reveal my secret. However, I still felt uncomfortable, but not because I was finally on a date with a man, but because I didn't want someone to see me with another man.

I continued to struggle with coming out, and before I knew it, I took a work assignment in China. Working in China was full on, but I still managed to go on runs during good air-quality days (which were very few). Ironically, the self-reflective

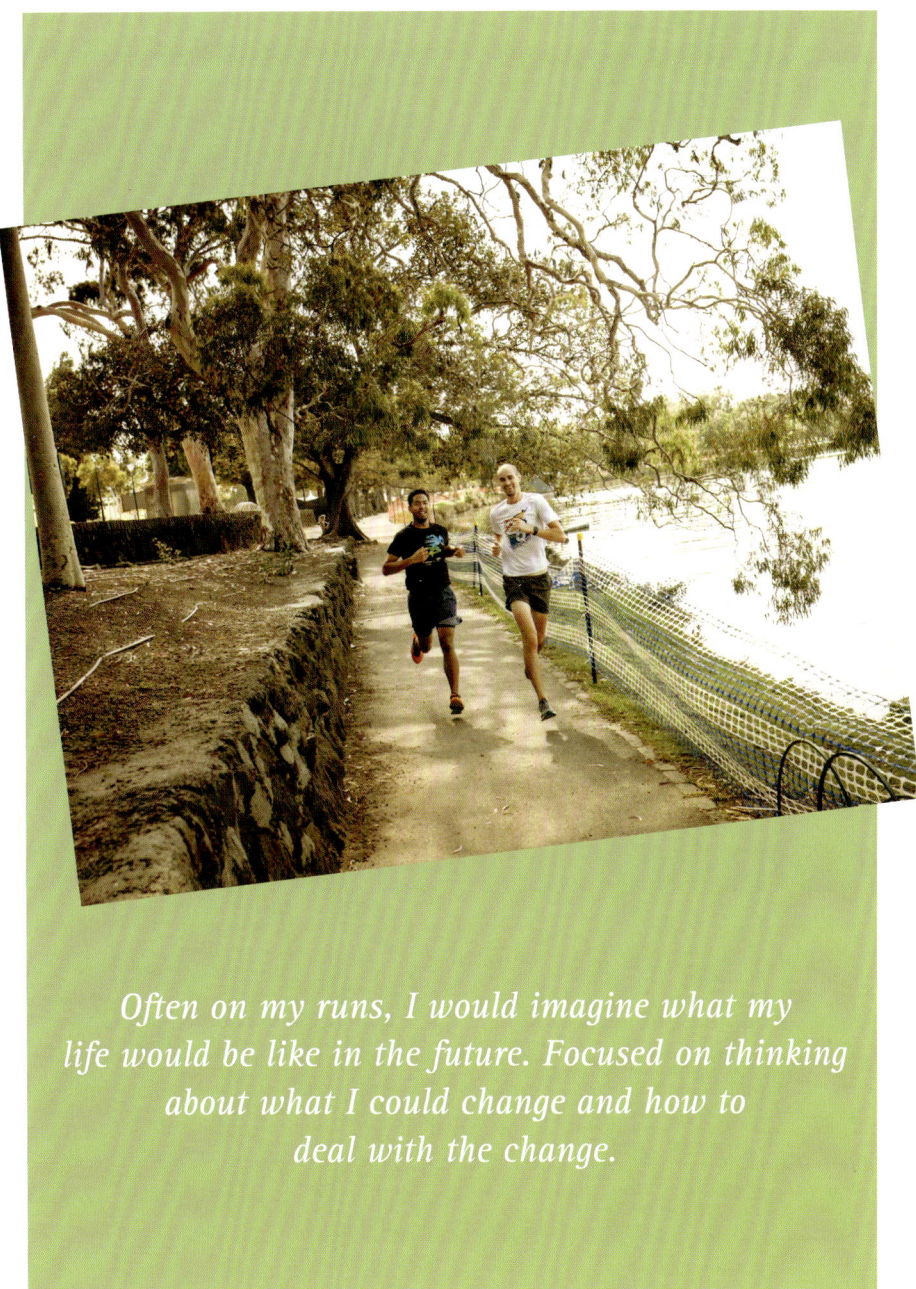

*Often on my runs, I would imagine what my
life would be like in the future. Focused on thinking
about what I could change and how to
deal with the change.*

loneliness that I sought in running slowly transformed to a fearful loneliness. Being surrounded by twenty-four million people in one city made me want to seek companionship. I wanted to be with and care for someone. That someone would be a man. After my first year in China, I decided to come out, first to a close friend and then to my family.

During my first work visit to China, I had a taste of what life in China would be like. I was staying in a hotel on the outskirts of Suzhou and the weather looked ripe for a run. I planned out a twelve-mile course around Jinji Lake, and about three quarters of the way, I had to stop; I could not breathe. I felt a tightness in my chest and experienced a dizzy spell. I had never experienced this feeling before, and later found out that the pollution index was well over 200 AQI for the day. My days of running in China would be limited and confined mostly to a treadmill.

When I moved to Shanghai, I tried running outdoors again. The key was to run very early in the morning when the city was asleep. It turned out to be one of the best ways to see Shanghai. Any visitor to China gets a taste of what 1.3 billion people feels like; it can be confronting and unnerving. But early in the morning, the city is for exploring.

I lived in the French Concession (which had some beautiful European-inspired architecture mixed with Chinese characteristics but was full of expats) and made it a point to run and explore the surrounding neighborhoods.

The early morning scents of street vendors preparing dumplings and porridge, cars and buses sitting lifeless on the road, and seeing the city "wake up," made my experience living in China truly special. Often during my runs, I would pass shopping plazas and parks and would see groups of older women known as "dancing grannies" doing various dance routines to the latest pop songs.

From time to time, I would run to The Bund (which I reserved for days when my body needed a reward) through the many small neighborhoods between my apartment and the Huangpu River. Seeing how the locals lived and running down almost empty tree-lined streets (that would normally be packed with cars, pedestrians, and bicycles) was an experience I never imagined in such a large city.

A good friend of mine and his wife had relocated to Beijing for work and invited me for a visit. I had been on an app communicating with an Australian guy named Johnny, who lived in Beijing, and I thought it would give me a good excuse to meet him in person.

We arranged to meet for a run in Olympic Park. When he arrived the next morning, he showed up with a "friend" and I was a bit confused. I wasn't sure what I had signed up for. A date? Or was he trying to set me up with someone else? We ended up running a 15k on one of the hottest days in Beijing, and when we arrived back at the subway stop, they both said goodbye and headed home. I wasn't exactly sure what had happened and wondered if I would ever hear from him again.

That evening during dinner with my friends, he sent me a text that said he had enjoyed the run and would like to meet up soon. We met for breakfast the next day and agreed that we would continue to meet up whether in Beijing or Shanghai.

We started commuting back and forth between Shanghai and Beijing, but I was getting ready to move back to the States. We decided to give long distance a try, and maybe Johnny would move to California in a year's time. Every day we would Facetime and we planned several trips, including one to New York to participate in the New York City Triathlon.

Finally, it was decided. Johnny would move to the States. Settling in to southern California, we picked up on our running time together and ultimately made the big decision.

In December 2018, my family and I flew to Melbourne, Australia, Johnny's hometown. We would be married on the thirty-first. The morning started with a group of friends running a 5k along the Yarra River. The ceremony was held at Glasshaus, a nursery inside of a rustic warehouse. Johnny surprised me with a choir that sang hymns throughout the ceremony.

We had oysters and champagne before walking our guests through the Royal Botanic Gardens, followed by a meal of Australian and Asian cuisine, which was a perfect way to represent our union. The most memorable part of the evening was when we gave our speech to the crowd of one hundred guests.

We joke about how we met and how we were able to find love through running. The love that we felt from everyone, being treated as equals, meant so much for the both of us.

There was a lot of laughter and tears that day, all ending with fireworks bursting across the city to ring in the new year. A chance date for a run in Beijing had led me to this point. It has been a marathon of another sort, but at last, I had crossed my own finish line. Or perhaps it was just the starting line.

Joe Suntharaphat: *Twenty Marathons . . . one ultra-marathons . . . three triathlons . . . ten states . . . two continents . . . Kilometers = limitless.*

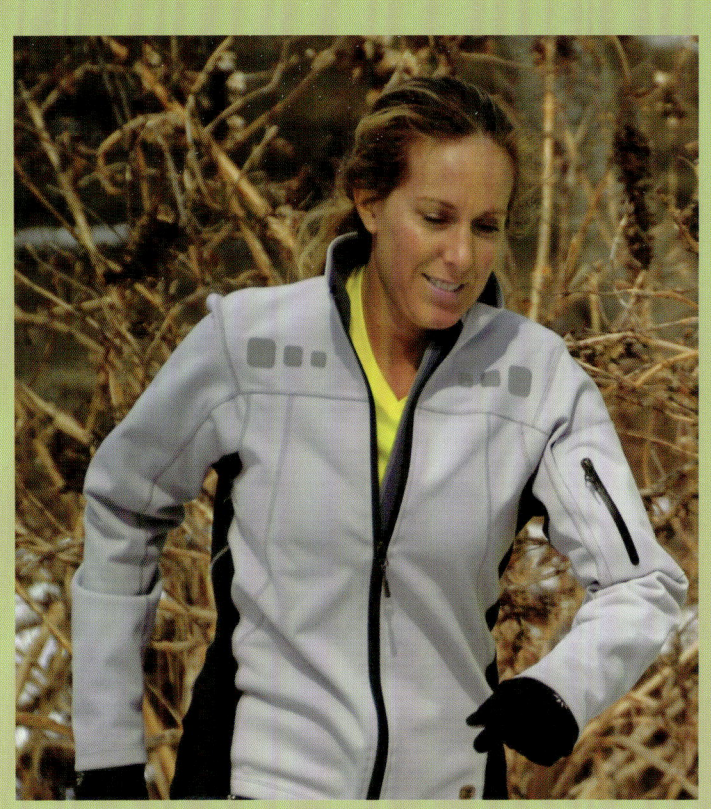

As a child, riding my bike alongside my father while he ran long distances was a regular occurrence.

Track Time with Dad

Ilse E. Abusamra

The high jump pit on the infield of a cinder track at a small private school in Massachusetts, where I often sprawled as a young child, was the first place I was introduced to running. The daughter of a longtime track and cross-country coach, I grew up surrounded by the sport. Many hot and humid summer evenings, my mother and I cheered for my father at local road races. As a child, riding my bike alongside my father while he ran long distances was a regular occurrence. Sometimes, our white German Shepherd even ran with us along quiet country roads. As an observer and one of the loudest cheerers around (I got that talent from my mother), perhaps I was destined to become a runner. But what I have gained from the sport has brought me to a far deeper place.

> *As an observer and one of the loudest cheerers around (I got that talent from my mother), perhaps I was destined to become a runner.*

My father, "the coach," didn't allow me to start running until eighth grade, as he was aware of the dangers of children being allowed to run distances at a young age. From his research and the seriousness with which he approached the sport, if I chose to enter the sport, he wanted me to start it at a time when I was both mentally and physically ready to both handle it and appreciate it. I dabbled with the sport as an eighth-grader doing cross-country and track, but my true dedication developed in high school. It was there where I experienced the meaning of team and accountability. Of course, as the coach's daughter, I felt both an obligation to try my best in all aspects of the sport, but also to respect it. I was lucky enough to find a group of peers with whom I connected, but that bond brought us so much more: it enabled us to charge through puddles with abandon, power up hills in freezing rain together, do repeat miles on muddy fields, and be tough when it counted. It certainly didn't hurt that I was part of an undefeated team that competed at the highest levels in our league and in New England. The drive and passion we developed were genuine. I was lucky enough to spend all four years of college running cross-country, indoor track and outdoor track, along with equally wonderful young women. Arriving at Motel 6 late on a Friday night, racing Saturday morning, and hopping in the vans to get back to our small Division III college campus in Maine was exactly where I wanted to be.

> ## *It was there where I experienced the meaning of team and accountability.*

When the time arrived that I had become faster and my father had slowed just a little, our paces were similar. And it was around the same time when my father made a deal with me: he would come out of his self-proclaimed "marathon retirement" if and when I qualified for the Boston Marathon. You see, when I was younger, my parents were teaching and taking care of a dorm on a private high school campus. In addition, my father was coaching most seasons and somehow finding time to get in his own running. After seriously training and competing in nine marathons, he decided that training simply took too much time away from my mother and me. But I had a sneaking suspicion that if I were lucky enough to qualify for Boston, he would resurface. He couldn't stay away. As if he had run a marathon just recently, when it had really been thirteen years prior, he didn't skip a beat. With ease, he ran a 3:28, qualifying for Boston with a twenty-two-minute cushion. Sadly, when Boston came around the following April, he was injured and unable to run, so we weren't able to run that marathon together.

As time went by, my father's running slowed a bit more due to creaky sacroiliac joints (though his passion and love for the sport continue to run strong!), and now he is often the one biking alongside me on my long runs. In the summers, when I spend the vast majority of my time at my parents' house, I will sometimes attempt to do long runs in the heat (a very challenging task for me). If my father isn't on the bike alongside me for one reason or another, often, as I come around a corner, he is there in the car with our German Shepherd and a cold energy drink to share. No matter if we are both running slowly together, or if my dad is on the bike or driving to meet me on various country roads, this shared experience of running is a huge joy for both of us.

As I have gotten older, the role of running in my life has shifted. It's now the time I spend with dear friends at 6 a.m. every morning in Central Park. We discuss politics, work, Broadway shows, new restaurants, and, of course, running. With these

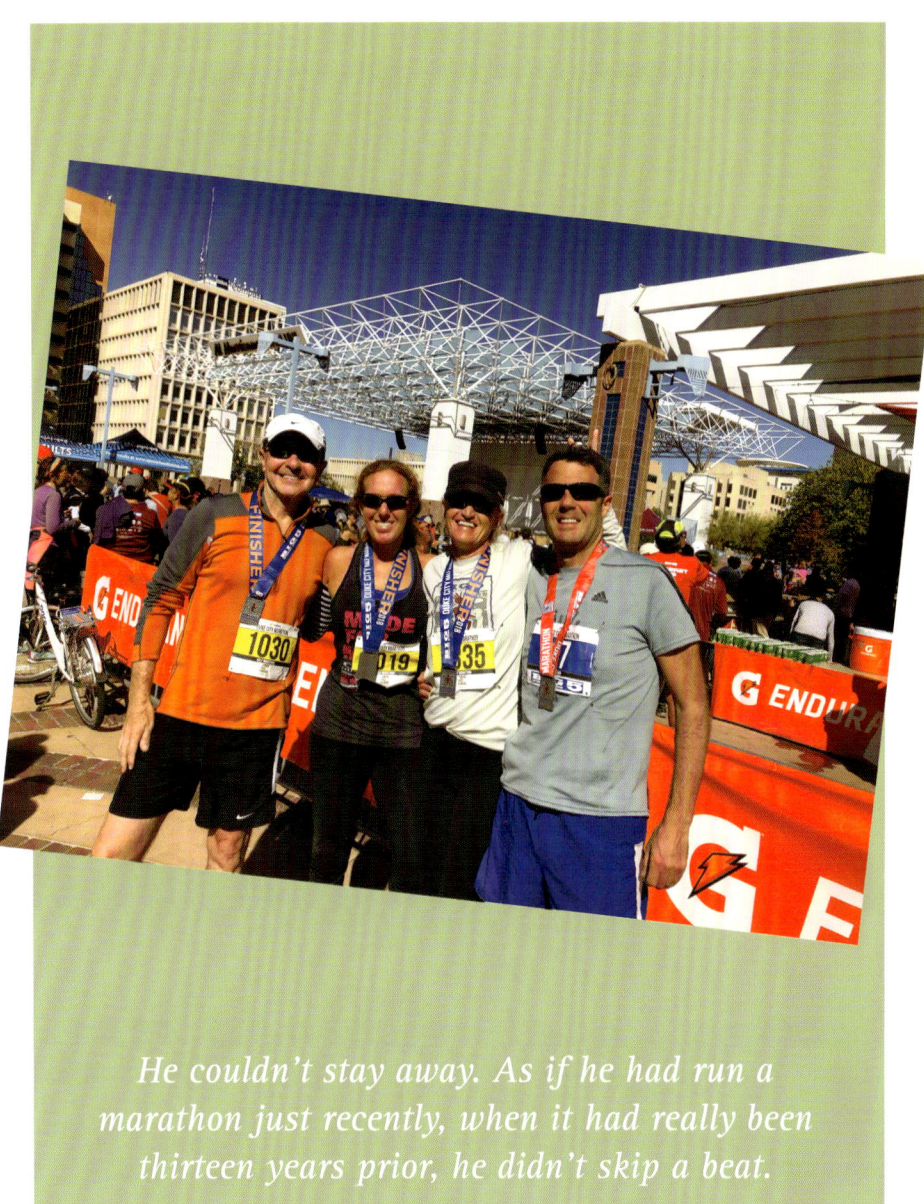

He couldn't stay away. As if he had run a marathon just recently, when it had really been thirteen years prior, he didn't skip a beat.

friends, I have traveled to multiple countries and states to run marathons. Beyond the connections I have with friends through the sport, it has also been a way for me to see more of the country and the world. There are few things better than running the Paris, Reykjavik, or Philadelphia Marathon surrounded by some of my best friends and our families. Everything has officially come full circle since my father, along with my mother, is now the one who is cheering me on at marathons around the world.

The tables have turned, but neither my dad nor I would have it any other way. Running has provided a backbone to my daily existence and a constant in my life. I have learned a great deal from the sport: responsibility, dedication, and respect for the distance, along with so much more. I run because I crave fresh air in my lungs and the opportunity to connect with treasured friends in the wee hours of the morning. I run for the challenge and the sense of accomplishment that I feel when I cross the finish line. I run for the rush of adrenaline that courses through my body after an especially hard race. I run to push my body and keep it working as it should. I run to explore different cities and countries as there is no better way to do that than on foot. I am often reminded of how my father has instilled that same love of running into countless high school runners. So many of his former runners still turn to him for advice, invite him to their weddings, and keep in touch regularly. As well, running still plays a large role in their adult lives, sometimes at a very high level. It is due to my father and his deep love of running that I have met many of my best friends and experienced many of my most satisfying moments. For that, I am deeply grateful.

After competing in high school and college, **Ilse Abusamra** *has run forty-two marathons and countless shorter races around the country and in Europe, many with her father and dear friends. She cherishes the time spent outdoors, the fresh air in her lungs, and all that she has learned from thousands of miles on her feet.*

The Mountain, Marathons, and Me

Keith LaScalea

Wouldn't it be a fun challenge to speed down 26.2 miles of the Mighty Rockies? The Revel Rockies Marathon, which starts in the Rocky Mountains and winds down to the foothills of Denver, could help me answer the question so many of us have asked ourselves.

I knew I wouldn't be winning this race, or any marathon for that matter, but that's never the point for us amateur runners. But could this marathon become my new PR? Runners are always striving to hit this hallowed goal, the personal record, and I hoped the downward course would help me achieve a new one.

This race reminded me again of just how remarkable the marathon is: a mix of glory and treachery. Marathons have helped me make new friendships and solidify old ones, share in the community of man, and enjoy some outstanding adventures as I've pursued my quest to run a marathon in all fifty US states. I have also been reminded of how tough enduring 26.2 miles is, how it continually beats on me, and how I have yet to actually master it.

We wound up the Colorado Mountains with runners from all over the west. A long-braided young Native American man from Wyoming sat beside me on the last bus up (strict departure time: 4:15 a.m.!). Though our lives were very different, we shared the same weary early-morning eyes as well as a common goal of success over the mountain. Running adventures are as much about seeing the varied landscapes as they are about meeting people whom I would not usually encounter in life.

Along my treks, I have met a lot of really interesting people, some who have never run a marathon and some who have completed the fifty-state-marathon circuit five times over.

Once on the way to a marathon in Tennessee, a delayed layover led to an evening in a pink limousine with a vivacious Ghanaian woman headed to a barbeque joint, followed by an unexpected trip to Graceland. I never could have expected such an interesting day when I woke up that morning. Another race, in Arkansas, led me to meet workers at an elephant sanctuary outside Little Rock and to better appreciate the important work they were doing with these majestic beasts.

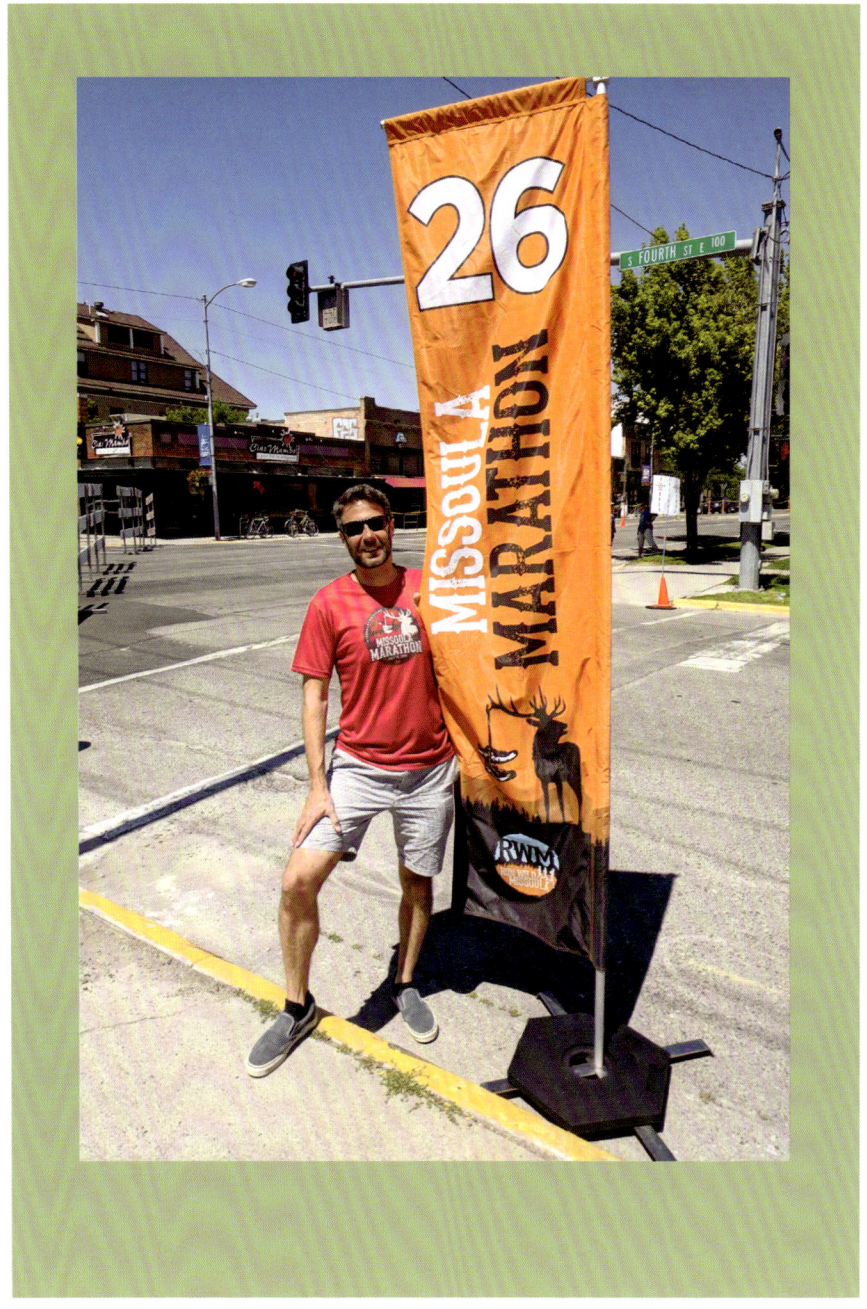

While running the Las Vegas Marathon, I met a runner dressed in a tutu who, with his "magic wand," offered us free wishes for better finish times. His spirit made the race a lot more amusing and made the miles pass more easily.

Once, at the end of a marathon, a kind soul saw me in my bedraggled state and offered to bring me a soda. I half-realized he was one of the other runners, though he looked like he was freshly showered and just out for a casual stroll. After a few sips of Coke and improved sensibility, I asked him if he had run one of the races that day. He modestly admitted he came in first place in the marathon—about an hour before me!

This race reminded me again of just how remarkable the marathon is: a mix of glory and treachery.

I started running marathons largely because I was inspired by the people streaming past my home each November. Runners of every shape, size, and color come together in a day that positively electrifies New York City. This spirit of excitement was also exemplified during the First Light Marathon. During this occasion in Mobile, Alabama, my soul was boosted while running alongside and meeting many of the adults with cognitive and physical disabilities who either walked, wheel-chaired, or were pushed by caretakers to the 26.2-mile finish line, where Southern belles dressed in ballgowns danced for us all. It was likely not by chance that we passed in front of the Alabama Institute for the Deaf and Blind along the course. Seeing the sheer joy in the expressions of all those finishing this race reminded me of how the marathon can uplift all of us regardless of innate ability. Marathons can be truly moving.

Marathons afford me the ability to see beyond my narrow scope of the world, and I gladly obey their calling. There is fun to be had with all these strangers as we fulfill our respective big dreams.

A chance conversation at the Berlin Marathon with a nearby American blossomed into an unlikely friendship. Sheila and her husband are farmers from South Dakota. We quickly realized she was on target to complete her hundredth marathon around the same time I might complete my fiftieth, so a trip to South Dakota the next year seemed reasonable. You can imagine my surprise when I entered my hotel room there to find it decorated with balloons and Happy Fiftieth signs! She arranged to break in before I arrived to show me real South Dakotan charm and a great marathon welcome. After the race was over, Shelia and Kevin let me drive their tractor, a real marvel of modern engineering, while sowing soybeans. I also had the opportunity to witness the amazing bands and community in their mega-church on the Sunday of my visit—a definite change from my usual weekend routine. We have continued to meet up and run together every year since.

Sometimes the marathon also allows you to re-cultivate old relationships. One of my happiest running moments occurred when my best childhood friend, Mike, completed his first marathon alongside me in an Atlanta park in the coldest January. At the end, we were embraced by his wife and kids with hugs that warmed our frozen bodies and strengthened our bonds. Tired, yet proud, we were able to look back on 26.2 miles and 35-plus years of friendship.

Marathons afford me the ability to see beyond my narrow scope of the world, and I gladly obey their calling.

Of course, the marathon can also be the centerpiece of any vacation. Traveling with close friends like Kenton, Mitch, Adam, and our families to the Shires of Vermont Marathon made for some vivid wet memories, as runners and cheerers alike were treated to brisk rains throughout the morning of our race. Of course, there was no shortage of family members who said yes to joining me for a trip to Paris for a marathon along the Seine. Another of my marathon-traveling pals, Phil, brings his beloved Bugs Bunny stuffed animal with him to each of our races as an amulet. Bugs was especially helpful to him, our friends Iron Maureen and Incredible Ilse, and me in Myrtle Beach, South Carolina, as we all sped quickly through our forty-degree races. Bugs is also a fan of all the friends who have rabbited me or who I have rabbited along in competitions: Bina, Michael B., Michael C., Sean, Kevin, Will, Emily, David, Peggy, and Meghan. Rabbiting friends along a course is yet another way we marathoners share the joys and pains of a race and make memories. I look forward to upcoming journeys with friends in Alaska and Hawaii, where the marathon will be a part of our holiday happenings.

Up, up, up we sailed through quaint mountain towns like Evergreen with road names like Squaw Pass. I was really surprised to see how many people lived so high in the sky, at well over a six-thousand-foot altitude, but I could understand why the beautiful alpine surroundings filled with crisp clean air would attract them far above the Mile High City. Also, the landscape clearly displayed why we marathoners felt compelled to find an adventure in running there.

Whether it be racing through the high deserts of Oregon, the gloriously golden autumnal forests around Richmond, the rolling landscapes of New England, or the Sand Hills of Nebraska, there is a moment in every race where I feel overwhelmed by the grandeur that is all around us. Paradoxically, the marathon forces us to slow down and attend to it. I will never forget the time my friend Andrea and I passed each other going in opposite directions over the Golden Gate Bridge during the San Francisco Marathon. Enshrouded in clouds, the bridge shielded our views of one another until the very last minute. A dreamy, mystical sensation came over me as I heard her voice call out to me and then dissipate quickly in the fog. The next few miles felt cushioned, buoyed by the beauty of the moment.

Another indelible marathon moment was during the Duke City Marathon in Albuquerque, New Mexico. About eight miles into the race, a multicolored hot air balloon sailed slowly up into the sky. I was dazzled and distracted from my run, but the delight only multiplied as another, and then another, and yet another balloon rose up high above us. Before long there were scores of balloons in the sky, blunting the image of 26.2 miles in my mind.

A dreamy, mystical sensation came over me as I heard her voice call out to me and then dissipate quickly in the fog.

There was a palpable collective sense of anticipation in all of us on the bus to the Rockies, since most of us had no idea what it would mean to traverse 26.2 miles straight down a mountain in the middle of a hot August summer. Nerves jittered, bladders twitched, and muscles began to awaken as we got closer to the starting point. What could we expect? Could we do this? It's moments of trepidation like these when I feel most connected to those around me. We run alone yet we runners share our battle with the distance. We each also come to confront ourselves—our bodies, our minds, and our souls. We are forced to realize our strengths and weaknesses in the most poignant ways possible. While the legs and the heart start strong, the distance has a way of whittling them down with every progressive step. The elements may work in our favor or we may suffer excess heat half way through. A course may be slippery and a fall is never impossible, as I learned during a marathon when I turned a corner too quickly, slipped on some pebbles, and was rewarded with a bunch of fractured ribs. Likewise, a sprained ankle in a pothole during the Baltimore Marathon made for a challenging last twenty-three miles. Hills and sharp turns conspire against us all. Pests may also throw us off course, as I found out when a yellow jacket bit me on the face during the Akron Marathon. Nevertheless, we line up and choose to put it all out on the road together and push forward as best we can, with the occasional course correction as needed.

Marathon running is truly a solo sport, but anyone who has run this distance will tell you that they feel propelled by all the others who run beside them. One of my most vivid memories of marathon comradery occurred as more than fifty thousand runners traversed the Verrazano Bridge from Staten Island to Brooklyn. Footfalls seemed to coalesce into a steady march. Like one giant super-organism moving in lockstep, the tempo of our collective beat called out to the world, "We are one; we do this together." There is no feeling quite like the exhilaration of realizing how connected you are to the thousands of humans around you, all racing toward a common goal. It's the ultimate insider moment!

The twisting, turning bus ride through these dark, early morning hours was unkind to my full bladder ("Don't forget to hydrate in the mountains," of course, being the mantra of this race as per my Denver hosts, Diana and David). My quick dismount from the bus to the woods caused me to miss the opportunity to apply sunscreen from the friendly, chatty, pig-tailed young woman sitting behind me—a mistake I would later regret after being assaulted by the hot, high-altitude Colorado sun, resulting in burned skin and chapped lips. But no matter, the start was before us, and it was only a momentary 3, 2, 1. . . GO!

Marathon running is truly a solo sport, but anyone who has run this distance will tell you that they feel propelled by all the others who run beside them.

I had been warned by my experienced running friends that downhills can be brutal, so I cautiously approached down-mountain. I was also concerned that the ten-thousand-foot altitude would slowly eat at me, especially since I had had only about thirty-six hours to acclimatize to the city far below us. But the cool, fresh early morning air was exhilarating. I felt strong and found my natural pace. Starting to pass a lot of other runners, I soon found myself in sight of the front-runners. I tried to slow a bit lest I burn out too quickly, but my sense of freedom in the picturesque scenery just let me fly. Green mountains with occasional pristine lakes and the sun rising over them inspired me.

Non-distance runners often wonder why we runners put ourselves through the travails of our sometimes-excruciating training and these long races. While the preparation definitely has its distinct challenges, it's all worth it for moments like this—when one feels the beauty of nature, of life, of the divine presented in full force up close. Combined with the truly breathtaking (in all its senses) nature of the runs, I never feel

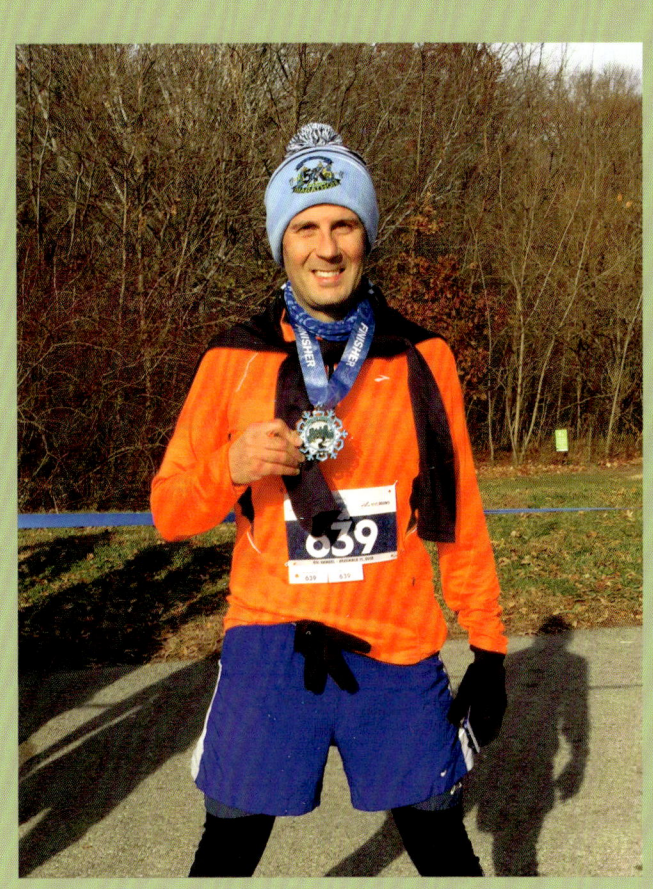

*I tried to slow a bit lest I burn out too quickly,
but my sense of freedom in the picturesque scenery
just let me fly.*

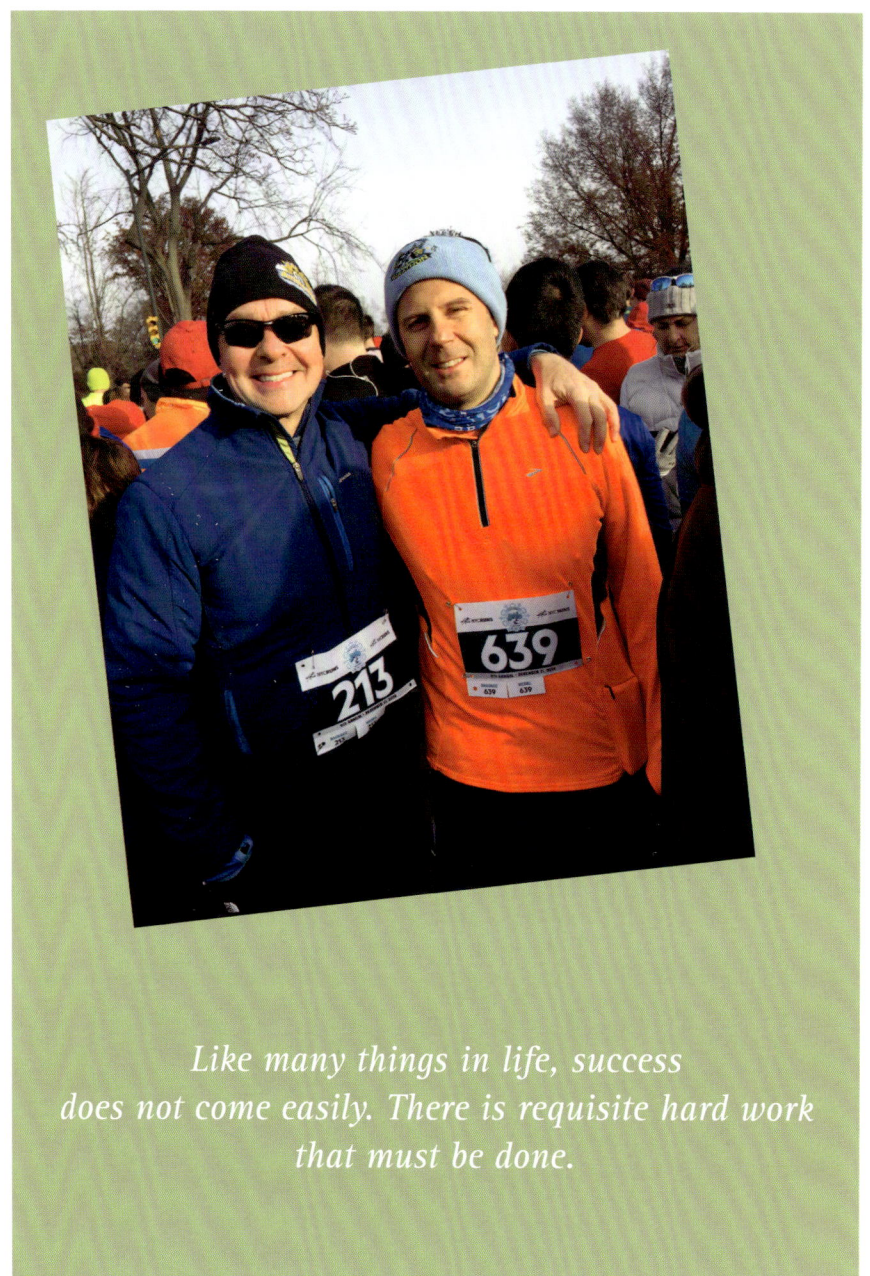

*Like many things in life, success
does not come easily. There is requisite hard work
that must be done.*

more alive than at moments like this. My Rocky Mountain High transcended all other thoughts, concerns, and worries, and my mind became filled with pure joy.

The good spirit kept up through the half way (13.1 miles) point. I knew I was going fast, but since there were no clocks on the course and I do not usually run with a watch, I did not know just how fast. Imagine my surprise to learn, after the race, that this was my fastest half marathon in years. Around mile fourteen, though, qualms started to creep into my brain, and my legs began to feel as heavy as concrete. I was able to push out the usual nasty this-is-too-hard-for-me thoughts for a while, reminding myself that I can accomplish this mountain mission. I had just the week before completed my personal forty-one-day-challenge to run every day. "You have fought this distance before," I repeated. It's like this at some point in every race—the typical refrain in my mind of self-doubt debating with the remembrance of the many miles run and races completed.

Like many things in life, success does not come easily. There is requisite hard work that must be done. I am not someone who takes shortcuts. Whether it be my schooling, training, or current work, I must push hard to keep pace with the others around me. I recount to myself the arduous groundwork I have put in to get here (pounding the pavement day after day; the grueling winter treadmill miles; and the occasional beach/ trail runs) and I try to convince myself I am prepared and strong enough to have a successful race. As though the race directors heard my inner dialogue, the mile markers along this course now had little positive messages connected to them and they began to galvanize me. My favorites include: "Chuck Norris can't do this," "You're sort of a big deal," "Pain is temporary. Pride is forever," and "One day you won't be able to do this. But that day is NOT today." The marathon calls us to keep training, keep pushing, and keep dreaming of big pursuits.

Push on, my brain insists. Just make it to mile fifteen . . . done. Get to sixteen and reassess . . . done. Soon I see the half marathoners (who started an hour later and half way down the mountain), and the sight of fresh runners at the start of their race revives me somewhat. Keep running to seventeen. . . okay, done. Have a Gu supplement, get to eighteen . . . done. But now I was ambling more slowly as the calves become heavier. At this point, the sun was higher in the sky and beginning to take its toll; gone were the sweet, cool breezes. I was probably at only about seven thousand feet by then, and it seemed the temperature warmed about twenty degrees. It was beginning to cook me.

At around mile eighteen, I heard a small pace group chasing behind me. I became a little panicked thinking it was the 3:30 folks. What a shock it was to me when I saw the pacer had 3:05 written on the sign stuck in his hat! I had never once run that fast to mile eighteen of a marathon. Maybe I could achieve that PR, after all. I was loving the speed of downhill running. Exhilarated about this, but with legs slowly turning to solid lead, I just could not keep up with this group. I watched them sprint ahead but considered I could still have a very good finish if only I keep it going to nineteen . . . twenty . . . twenty-one . . . My mind turned to my favorite church billboard of all time: "They shall run and not grow weary," carefully selected to motivate marathoners in Kansas City, Missouri's race.

I've often been asked what I think about during a long run, and I can accurately say there is a relatively consistent pattern of elation followed by near-crushing insecurity that I still have not conquered during a marathon (one would think by state number thirty-sesven, this should have been easy for me). This is followed by multiple assessments of why. Why am I wimping out? Why can't I keep up the pace? Why won't my body cooperate? Why is my mind not stronger at pushing out the uncertainty? Why am I feeling so hot? Why did I just drink two cups of Gatorade instead of one? Why did Windsor Castle need to be so far from the start, making this race so long? Why do I just want to walk? How annoying to be plagued by all these questions! The tired brain could only handle one of these at a time, much like the legs could only run one step at a time. "Focus," the brain yelled out. "Just get to the next mile and keep moving. Notice the splendor around you. Ignore the fatigue. Ignore the pain. Soon you will be able to rest."

> ### *"Just get to the next mile and keep moving. Notice the splendor around you. Ignore the fatigue. Ignore the pain. Soon you will be able to rest."*

Leaden legs swiftly turned to osmium as I spotted the mile-twenty marker. My brain reassured me that I have covered more than the remaining miles even on easy training days. "You can do more than this in your sleep," I repeated to myself. The mind eased a little as I crept into the last 6.2 miles, but the lower body continued to resent me. I found myself walking the distance from the full marathon markers to the half marathon markers, a tenth of a mile further along, hating myself the whole time for slowing so much. There are few miseries worse than watching runners passing me and realizing my place is progressively worsening. Now the disillusioned soul and the wingless legs were in consort against the heart that was still holding out hope for a respectable finish time . . .

The ongoing pain reminded me I was alive—alive and still ready to take on the challenge of the marathon. Some authors have posited we are born to run, that our lives are evolved to be able to escape. Many a songwriter has articulated the connection between pain and heightened awareness. Perhaps it is my primitive mammalian brain sending out endorphins to combat the suffering that brings my runner's high. Maybe it's the fatigued brain tuning out all the inconsequential matters of life, and focusing me on the here and now, on the essential priorities of my mind, body and spirit. I am not quite sure why, but few things in life can motivate like this. It is yet another way the marathon calls me back.

All my senses are continually piqued during these mammoth sessions. Watching the flamboyant New Orleans festivities surrounding the Mardi Gras Marathon excited my spirit. Listening to the multitude of Americana bands on the course of the Marine Corps Marathon in Washington, DC stirred my patriotic soul. Feeling the sunlight on my skin as I ran in and out of the resplendent caverns in St. George, Utah, warmed my core. Smelling the scent of light spring rains while running through Churchill Downs ahead of the Kentucky Derby rekindled happy adolescent memories of working with horses. Tasting the have-these-ever-been-so-delicious-in-my-life orange slices during my sunny Boston Marathon sweetened my steps to the end of this historic race. Is it any surprise we marathoners feel so alive during a race?

The last few miles were marked with a few slight uphills, which I was surprisingly happy to see. Mile twenty-one came, as did eventually twenty-two. A year and a day ensued until mile –twenty-three—only 3.2 miles to go. "Just keep going," I reproached. The aid station folks kindly cheered us ahead as they watched us limp through. Twenty-four came slowly, but I knew this would soon be done. It took me an eternity to get to mile twenty-five, but the last 1.2 miles were happily a bit better. Somewhere along the way the 3:15-, 3:25- and 3:35-pace groups all sped ahead of me, disenchanting me with each step. At mile twenty-six, the 3:40-pacer pulled ahead of me, but luckily the mind started to conquer the legs and I was able to keep step with the pacer. I passed her just before the finish line. (The pacer, of course, was not upset since she is supposed to finish at 3:40 and hopes to see competitors do the best they can.). A sweaty 26.2 miles done and medal draped across my chest, finally the finish line was behind me. The finish line always provides a chance to take a deep breath and recollect my senses.

The treachery of it! An amazing race time, my blessed PR, had been within my grasp, but it slipped away in the last eight miles. Despite my planning, the mountain got me in the end. I was sacrificed and subdued by it. My knees almost collapsed under me a few times, as soon as post-race mile 26.3. Walking was more of a struggle than at the end of any prior race. I better felt the pain most runners experience when completing a marathon, especially their first one. The aching from this one was historical for me. The mountain kept echoing in my muscles for days to come. Sitting, standing, walking, even taking baby steps became quite a feat, especially with my sunburned skin and lips. I had never felt this old. Yet the endorphins, in peak form, helped me to more fully appreciate my youth.

My mind becomes a clunky mix of both the demons and wonderful inspirations at the end of each long race. Luckily, like most humans who quickly forget pain, I am left with a net positive consideration of the whole affair. Though, I am almost always left wishing I could have pushed through just a little faster and a bit better. That is another reason I keep coming back. The mountain schooled me but also steadied me for the next adventure. The questions posed are now less arduous. When is the next marathon? What journey will call to me? Who will I get to know racing beside me? Where in this wonderful world will it be? And, how will I and my other marathon adventurers do battle again?

*I am not quite sure why, but few things
in life can motivate like this. It is yet another way
the marathon calls me back.*

I sat in the post-race area for a while along with the runners who ended before me, with my thoughts, happily watching other runners stream across the finish line. Once again, we were united—but on the other side of the race now. I saw the braided man and the pig-tailed woman cross over, as well as many others who I passed along the course. Some were first-time competitors who could now proudly claim "marathoner" as no longer an aspiration, but instead as achievement. Like comrades in arms, we were bonded. In fact, many were already crafting their war stories as they discussed their experiences with this marathon. I was content to be with them and to have completed my Colorado race.

But disappointment is also a common partner after any marathon. For most, it means the culmination of many months of effort. With the dream done, many are unsure where to go from there. For me, the answer is always clear, because within hours of completing a race, I am already considering the next one and planning a stronger attack plan. Like a junkie coming down from his high, I understand this might not be the healthiest behavior, but the marathon keeps beckoning me. Like a siren, it spotlights its spectacles and downplays its disadvantages. I'll have my chance to overcome the discontents next time. After all, there are far worse addictions one could possess than the marathon.

In the end, I was grateful to have the health and good faculties to go to battle with the mountain at all. I was pleased to have had such a good first 13.1 miles, and I was emboldened to train harder so that the second half of the next marathon would not continue to overpower me. I did not get that PR I was pining for, but it was all fine. I had completed another contest and was all the stronger for it. I answered my question: the mountain was a definite marathon challenge that yet again recapped how we runners need to calibrate our bodies, our minds, and even our souls for its rigors. One day, I might be stronger than The Marathon; it just wasn't this day.

Keith LaScalea *has run thousands of miles in his lifetime in races of all lengths, but it is the marathon that most mesmerizes him. He has completed more than sixty marathons to date with the goal of completing one in each of the United States. He writes about the love-hate relationship he has had with all those miles.*

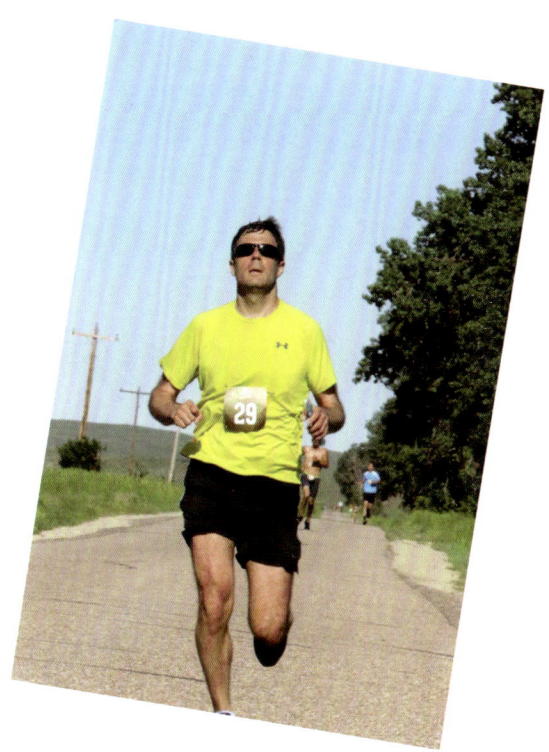

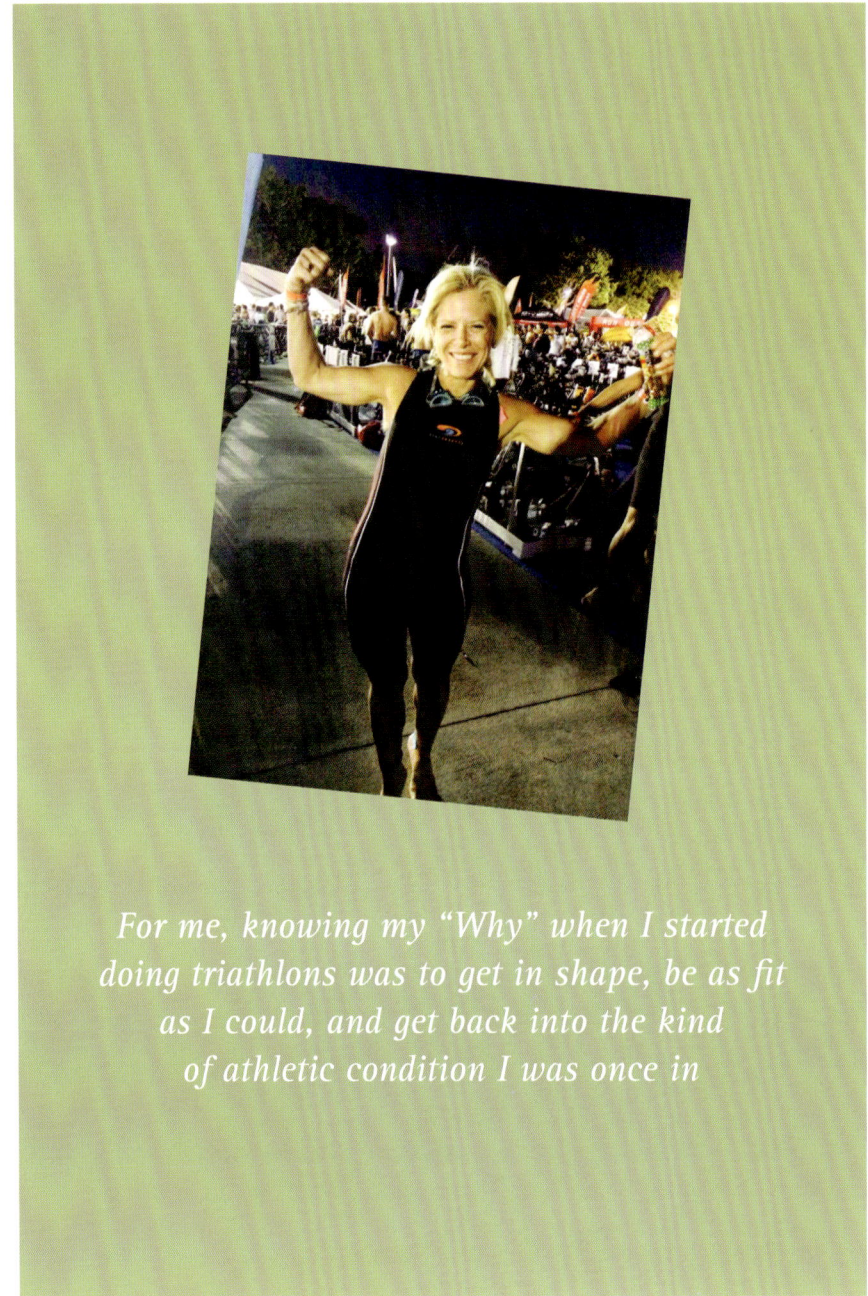

For me, knowing my "Why" when I started doing triathlons was to get in shape, be as fit as I could, and get back into the kind of athletic condition I was once in

Know Your Why

Lucy Danziger

You always have to know your "Why?"

Jillian Michaels taught me this during our cover story when I was the editor-in-chief of *SELF*, and we shot her four times for the cover, once every spring at the kick off of the "get back in shape" time of year, and each time she and I became better friends. Hers is a philosophy I admire: *Know your Why!* She would ask the contestants on *The Biggest Loser*, and once they had told her "I want to dance with my grandchildren," or whatever it was, she would play it back to them to motivate them to push through that tough workout or to successfully avoid the platter of donuts on the kitchen table as temptation. "Do this so you can dance with your grandchildren!" she'd yell at them, and it worked.

For me, knowing my "Why" when I started doing triathlons was to get in shape, be as fit as I could, and get back into the kind of athletic condition I was once in—before kids, before a big stressful desk job, before life and eating mindlessly led me to pack on the pounds in my early forties. So, at forty-five, I started eating healthy, motived also by my dad's heart disease and multiple scares, and I cut out all the bad stuff: cheese and fries and sweets and stupid chips or other junk food. Bye, cookie dough; bye, nightly drinking; bye, breadbasket. Very quickly I lost twenty, then twenty-five pounds, in what felt like no time, though it was about four months. As I got lighter, I also got faster and started to do better at triathlons; every finish, I found myself on the podium—meaning finishing within the top three spots in my age group. (In races all over, the competitors are grouped in divisions of five years, allowing you to feel good about your relative standing.)

I set my sights higher, started racing not just in New York but also in Florida and California, and longer distances—Olympics and then half-IRONMAN events—and though I didn't get faster, I could go farther and have fun training with a team of athletes half my age who were all talented at either running or biking or swimming, and a handful were really good at all three. My strength was my bike, but I could run fine. The swim was like watching a mouse churn butter: all arms and splash but little forward movement. I took lessons and showed up at the pool and told myself not to be humiliated when people passed me in the lane. They hit your feet and then go around you, and it was a shock at first—this whack on the bottom of the sole of my foot. But then I learned to expect it, and it all was just part of the fun of learning and challenging myself. I parked my ego at the pool deck door.

For me, knowing my "Why" when I started doing triathlons was to get in shape . . .

Then suddenly, the year I was turning fifty, everyone on the team decided to do an IRONMAN—either Lake Placid or Zurich—and, swept up in the idea that this could be a moment to try this crazy sounding distance, I signed up. I had no idea what I was getting myself into. I asked my family for "time" as my birthday gift: I needed to have the time to go to the pool in the mornings or evenings after work, to bike on Saturdays and run on Sundays, and prepare myself for a race to end all races. I sat the kids and my husband down at the kitchen table and explained my Why: to challenge myself in a way I never thought I could. "I would love your support." They nodded. But none of us had a clue what any of it really meant. I thought I would have to train about twelve to fourteen hours a week. It turned out to be more like sixteen, on top of a demanding job and travel schedule. But they were teenagers and away at school by now, so really it was my husband who had to cope with my absence. Luckily, I married a very independent guy who seems to love me, and for that I'm grateful!

The race is a 2.4-mile swim, and even after hours in the pool and stroke clinics, endless videos and drilling to get my forward glide to happen, I couldn't swim very fast. My signature was sinking between strokes, hula-hooping my hips in the water instead of staying streamlined, and not getting very far for the effort. So, it would be a long day. I didn't care. You have to get out of the water in under 2 hours and 20 minutes or you can't continue the race, and I managed to do it in 1 hour and 20. Then you bike 112 miles, and while I love to bike, that was going to be a long ride by any standards: I completed it in about a 6 hours and 30 minutes. Then you get off your bike and run a marathon. That part seemed most ridiculous, even to those of us who had run marathons, since most of the time you do this rested, on a fully fueled body, not after eight hours of exertion. But it also weirdly made sense. I thought of it as four loops around the lake, and just started running. And before too long, and before it got dark, I was rounding the corner on the final chute and seeing my time of under 13 hours. I was psyched when the announcer called out: "Lucy Danziger, you are an IRONMAN!" Then a little while later, after walking around and feeling light-headed, I got up to go see my friend finish and the next thing I knew, I had fainted. I had not had enough salts and my body just shut down. After a quick IV to replace my salts, I was back walking around. But even so, it was a euphoric experience and I thought: one and done. That was fun.

I missed the training. Turns out, I found hours on the road biking to be a Zen-like experience, a moving meditation that meant I could think and let the wind sweep away my stress as the bike carried me past beautiful wooded scenery all around New York City and up the Hudson River. So once I had finished that race, which I remembered fondly for its gloriously beautiful swim in pristine Lake Zurich and impressive vistas from the alpine climbs that made you want to burst into song ("The hills are alive . . ."), and then the flat and crowd-supported run around the lake, I actually thought: why not do another?

My first race Why was to be able to go through life knowing I had actually done an IRONMAN, and that motivation fueled me and stoked my training days. I treated myself to a nice hotel in Zurich and realized this was the ultimate fiftieth birthday present to myself. It was both indulgent, time-wise, and expensive (the bike alone costs thousands of dollars, plus the travel, the wetsuit, the training and coaching hours, the swim access—I don't want to think about the amount of money I spent). On some selfish level, I told myself this was a way of investing in myself and separating my aging process from my parents' generation—many of whom regarded turning fifty as the beginning of the end. It was what I call the "unimpeachable" excuse, meaning no one can fault you for being healthy!

My first race Why was to be able to go through life knowing I had actually done an IRONMAN, and that motivation fueled me and stoked my training days.

But in fact, the entire endeavor of training for IRONMAN distance racing is selfish. Still, that first race in Switzerland was a gift and a treasured memory: I loved that day, every hour of the nearly thirteen it took me to complete the race felt fueled by my Why. When I finished, I collapsed, literally fainted, but it was all worth it.

Then once I had finished my first IRONMAN, the question was: Why do it again? There was one simple answer: to try to qualify for Kona. Kona is the big one, the IRONMAN Championships that you can watch on television every fall, that shows the toughest course and the hardest of stories—humanity overcoming our limits to push through even after life's challenges like cancer or illness, injury or loss. The stories are beyond inspiring, and I thought: Everyone knows I do triathlons, from the people I work with to the most distant Facebook friend, and when the subject comes up, they always ask me, "The one in Hawaii?" and I have to answer: "No, the other ones." Like they are lesser ones. In a sense, they are, because to get to Kona you can't just pay your way in (other than an exorbitant charity slot). To be allowed to show up for that race, you have to qualify. In my age group, women fifty and over, that means you had to win your division. There is generally only one spot per race. (Sometimes the winner turns it down and the second finisher gets it, but that's a rare day.) Most of the fastest women in my age group would have beaten the heck out of me in sports in school. They are often former varsity track or swim stars. And I never would have even been on the same track or in the pool with them in college or high school; they are talented, where I just try hard. My crowning athletic achievement had been to be in the best boat in crew in high school, hardly the stuff of legends. But nonetheless, I wanted to try to compete at the highest levels. It was folly!

I loved that day, every hour of the nearly thirteen it took me to complete the race felt fueled by my Why.

I set my sights on Germany, the IRONMAN race in Frankfurt, because the team had chosen it. I had done Zurich blissfully unaware of the alpine climbs on the bike or the hot temps that threated to make the swim too warm to wear wetsuits. In the end, we could wear them—a major benefit to us non-swimmers since they allow you to float higher in the water and resist the drag or sinking with every stroke—so I figured just sign up and go. Don't overthink it, I told myself. I didn't, but I did over-train for it.

Frankfurt turned out to be another story: a tale of monsoon rain and wind gusts that whipped around buildings and knocked over small riders, like the 120-pound women who would be walloped so hard and fast that she went over like a toy soldier knocked down by an invisible hand—the officials dubbed these "single-rider crashes." Other than the weather, a more ominous problem had cropped up: I had been overtraining on my long runs, doing more mileage than my body could tolerate. Prior to my first race, the longest run I had completed was sixteen miles, which is less than most people do for a marathon. For this one, I did several of those and a twenty-miler. Most new triathletes build their fitness on the bike and don't do as many long runs as a marathoner—the downside of potential injury outweighs the upside of gaining fitness. You need to listen to your body and not run through the pain. When a sharp cutting, slicing pain crops up that feels like stabbing or burning crops up, that's your signal to dial it back.

I started landing funny, with a sharp pain in my left fore-foot, and sought out the counsel of a doctor who told me I likely had a "stress injury" and sent me to get an X-ray. It was inconclusive, so he sent me to get an MRI, but instead of looking at the film, he read the report, and it didn't pick up the fracture—which is common, I later found out. Too late. I booked my flight, stayed off the runs, and just gave myself a long taper of two weeks no running until the race. When I was "cleared for takeoff," my husband said to me: "You hear what you want to hear. Your doctor told you that you could race but you knew otherwise." Of course, he was right. After training for nine months, I didn't want to let go of the dream, though at this point I knew in my heart this would not go well. I had also managed to give myself a terrible "road rash" in a crash on Route 27 out in Long Island while training, so my left arm was bandaged and oozing, my foot was sore and hurting at every step. I got to Germany as the storm clouds gathered—the weather turning dark and mean-looking in every direction—and I thought, *If I could back out now, I would.* Still I kept on, which turned out to be stupid. But I was too far into this to back out now. My why had changed from trying to qualify for Kona to completing what I had started.

The team went to a pre-race event the afternoon before the race, and we all got to have a picture and moment at a book signing with Macca (Chris McCormack), then the number-one male triathlete in the world, who I had previously interviewed at *SELF* because of his involvement with raising money and awareness around breast cancer, a disease his mother died of. I told him about my foot, the pain at every step, and that I was here and would race and see what the day would bring. I thought he would tell me to bail. Instead he said: "It's going to suck either way, with or without the foot pain. . . . Embrace the suck!" he told me. He even wrote it as his autograph on a poster he gave out to participants. That night, I danced around the hotel room as I laid out my gear, trying to make light of the injury and the weather and the impending pain I would have to endure for 13 or so hours the next day: *Embrace the suck*, I told myself. This was going to suck.

The next day, hair braided as usual, gear on, and water bottle full of electrolytes, I showed up at the race under dark skies, and it was a miserable day from the minute I put on my wetsuit and got into the dark lake, which looked like an industrial runoff pool. No clear water here, like Zurich; instead it was dark and murky and, unlike in Switzerland, where the women and men started separately and merged on the course 500 meters out and were nicely spaced out from one another, here the men (mostly European) got into the water with us few women, and from about the fifth stroke, I was being pushed down into the water by large male arms that were trying—like me—to find a little open water to swim in. The first time one large male athlete pushed me under, I assumed it was a mistake—*he was just trying to find his stroke space*, I told myself as I tried to not panic and come up for air. But then as I came up spluttering, he did it again—his large hand on the middle of my back pushing down and—*WHAM*—down I went again, under the surface. I saw his legs kicking away as he swam over me, and now I was pissed. With both my hands, I yanked his ankle as hard as I could. "Watch where you're going!" He momentarily turned back to say something to me that I assume was German for *What the f–?* And I just said: "We're all in it together!"

But it felt like we were all out there alone. On the cold, windy, wet bike course, we did two loops: the first was like a summer carnival, with beer-drinking locals lining every foot of the course, singing and dancing and letting us know how happy they were we had come to Frankfurt to race. The second loop, some three hours later, there was no one there. I felt like I was digging deep to find the motivation. Why was I doing this again? Certainly not to get to Kona. I couldn't find my usual mojo. My foot hurt even on the bike. At this point, I would be lucky to finish and not come in last. It was going to be a long day. But I was here, and in it, and I vowed to finish.

Embrace the suck, *I told myself.* *This was going to suck.*

By the time I got off the bike and looked at my foot, it was swollen to twice its normal size. This had never happened before, and I was perplexed, since a bike shoe is rigid, the bottom made of a light, molded plastic almost like a ski boot. How was my foot so beat up? I shoved it into my running shoe in transition, knowing this would not be my day to qualify for Kona. At this point, I was behind my time goal by almost an hour. I had chosen to be cautious in the wind, having seen a woman right in front of me go down when a side gust whipped around a building and knocked her over, so I stayed out of my aero-bars and held on, white-knuckled, just to stay upright. At this point, I wasn't racing so much as covering the distance. As I set out on the run, I saw my coach, who said, "Quit now." I told him, "Look, either way it's going to be a long recovery. I might as well finish. I won't be able to run for six weeks; I can get through the next four to five hours."

My Why was rapidly changing: instead of trying to "qualify" for Kona, my new Why was: Don't be a quitter. Finish what you started, and don't come home with excuses. The run along the river entailed a few scrubby patches, and on one of these, I stepped on a small pebble, right at the point of my stress fracture, and it felt like my foot had been struck by a lightning bolt from the ground up. I knew what had happened: I had popped open the stress fracture, and the foot now was so painful—the tiny metatarsal bone shattered to pieces—that I could only land on my heel for the next eleven miles. But this wasn't something I would be able to see till later on the X-ray that showed my tiny foot bone in shards, like logs on a river all floating alongside each other. I started stepping gingerly, heel only, just to keep moving. Only about six miles to go, but it was getting dark. The race would be called at fifteen hours, two less than the usual cut off of seventeen hours, because in Frankfurt, the city residents didn't like the finish line noise lasting till midnight. So, if you didn't get to the line by 10 p.m., you could not call yourself a finisher, or be officially counted as an IRONMAN.

With my stomach reacting badly to all the gels and goo and possibly also to the stress of the pain, I started having what athletes euphemistically call "gastro distress," and with about three miles to go, I was literally having to decide between finishing the race in time to qualify as an IRONMAN or stopping to go to the bathroom. That could be a long stop, given the nature of my discomfort. I didn't know how far I had to go. At the side of the path, I saw an ambulance and medical tent and I asked a medic, *How far to the finish line?* He said five kilometers. I did some quick math. I had about fifteen minutes to go before the cut off, and even if I ran a five-minute mile, which I couldn't on my best day or most fit, this was not enough time to make it. I hoped he was wrong and decided to ignore that information. I could see the finish line on the other side of the river and hear the noise of the announcer, calling out "Mikael, you are an IRONMAN!" I still had one more out-and-back loop along the river to go, then I had to get over to the other side and enter the finish chutes. I had to go out a mile, and back a mile. I hobbled faster.

It was going to be a long day. But I was here, and in it, and I vowed to finish.

At this point, it was dark. The route looked like an abandoned parade littered with cups, everyone folding up their tables and chairs and heading home. We scattered athletes, mostly walking, were the last few to come in. I passed one super-fit male athlete who was walking. I asked what was wrong. He said: "Knee." I said, "Come on, come on, come on, you can do it. We gotta make the cutoff." He started running with me, baby steps, just to keep moving. As we finished the last mile with just minutes to go before the cutoff, I swept up all the athletes walking in, who had given up by now, telling them: "We gotta keep going, we can make the cutoff. Come on, come on, come on! You want to be an IRONMAN, you have to finish!" About seven of us were in this group as we approached the last block to the finish line. We were all well past the point of embracing the suck. We looked like an army returning from war, having lost. I kept hobbling, and suddenly I realized the medic was wrong, the finish was closer than he'd thought: about half a mile, then a few hundred yards. I finished in plenty of time: nearly ten minutes to spare. How the math was wrong in my head, I never did figure out.

About the time that I finished, I realized I had also messed up my bike shorts. Let's leave it at that, but it was truly gross. I had not wanted to stop to deal with it. I went into the showers in a trailer at the finish line area and took my pants off and put them in one shower and myself in another. A young woman was showering in a nearby stall, and I said: "Stay away from that shower," pointing to my bike shorts on the floor. She was pretty cheerful so I asked: "Did you make it?" No, she told me. She had had two flats and missed the cutoff by a minute. Heartbreaking. "Well, you're still an IRONMAN to me," I told her. But in the books, it didn't count officially. I realized then how lucky I was, or how stubborn, or perhaps how vain to have sets my sights so high in the first place. But I hadn't quit.

I figured out that I may not ever have the bragging rights of going to Kona, but I also had done what I set out to do. Finished. My next IRONMAN (yes, I had to redeem myself) was better, in New York City running through another injury, a partial hamstring tear, but in about twelve hours and twenty-five minutes. My perfect race eludes me. Going to Kona may be a dream unrealized, but I know this: I can finish what I start. I can embrace the suck, and I can learn more about myself on the road than anywhere else. In the times in my life when I nearly get defeated, pushed to my limits and challenged beyond what I think is my limit, I remember that I can run on a broken foot and finish a marathon in lightning white pain. I looked at the river that day and thought: *I would rather jump in it than not finish.* I would not come home with excuses. I did not want to set an example to my kids of quitting. Instead, I came home with a shattered foot and crutches, had to have a boot, then a cast, and a good four months of not running. I had one of those kneeling scooters where you steer yourself around your home like a kid, but your foot is propped on a padded cushion. To other people it all seemed a little nuts. Actually, it did to me as well. That wasn't so great for my family. But I knew what I could accomplish, and I didn't have to prove it to anyone else ever again. A footnote: after completing a third IRONMAN in New York IRONMAN the following year, I tried for my fourth IRONMAN at Lake Placid and didn't ever have a clear Why.

I had done well enough at New York to hold my head up high. Again, at Placid, I was injured—with a partially torn peroneal tendon in my left ankle, from rolling to the outside as I trained on the roads of Long Island, where the bread-loaf shape forces you to land slightly slanted to one side or another. I entered Placid in pain, and halfway through the marathon, after surviving another downpour on the bike and lightning during the swim (they pulled people out who had not started the last loop for home), I decided: races are not supposed to kill you. Or even injure you or leave you so broken you can't function.

I stopped at mile 13.1, after one loop that brought us back in town, and told myself: You don't have to finish. My Why was to be healthy, not end up in a boot and unable to run or play sports or even move around at work and on weekends. I wanted to have a life. I got back to my original Why: to be the fittest and healthiest I could be. I didn't want to do irreparable damage to my injured leg and never be able to run properly again. So, I decided to go to town after that half marathon and eat lunch and not be sad or despondent about it. I called my husband and he said, "It's just a race. There are lots of races. So what? You dropped out. No big deal. Don't make it bigger than it is." As usual, he was right. My Why is to be healthy and happy, and it was my choice. It's just a race. There are many of those, but you only have one body. Know your why and you will always do what you need to reach your goals. And be healthy out there!

Lucy Danziger *is the former editor-in-chief of* SELF *magazine, founder and CEO of* Hinted, *and a three-time IRONMAN finisher. She has never qualified for Kona and probably never will. And that is okay with her.*

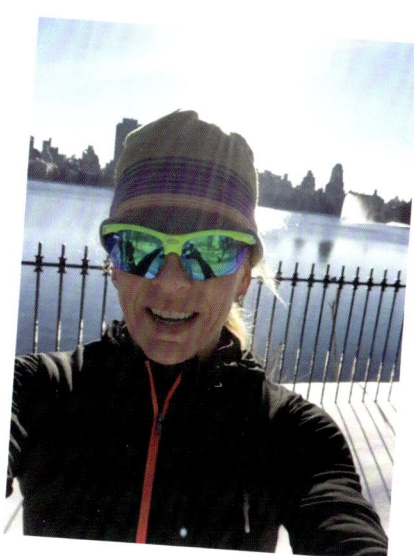

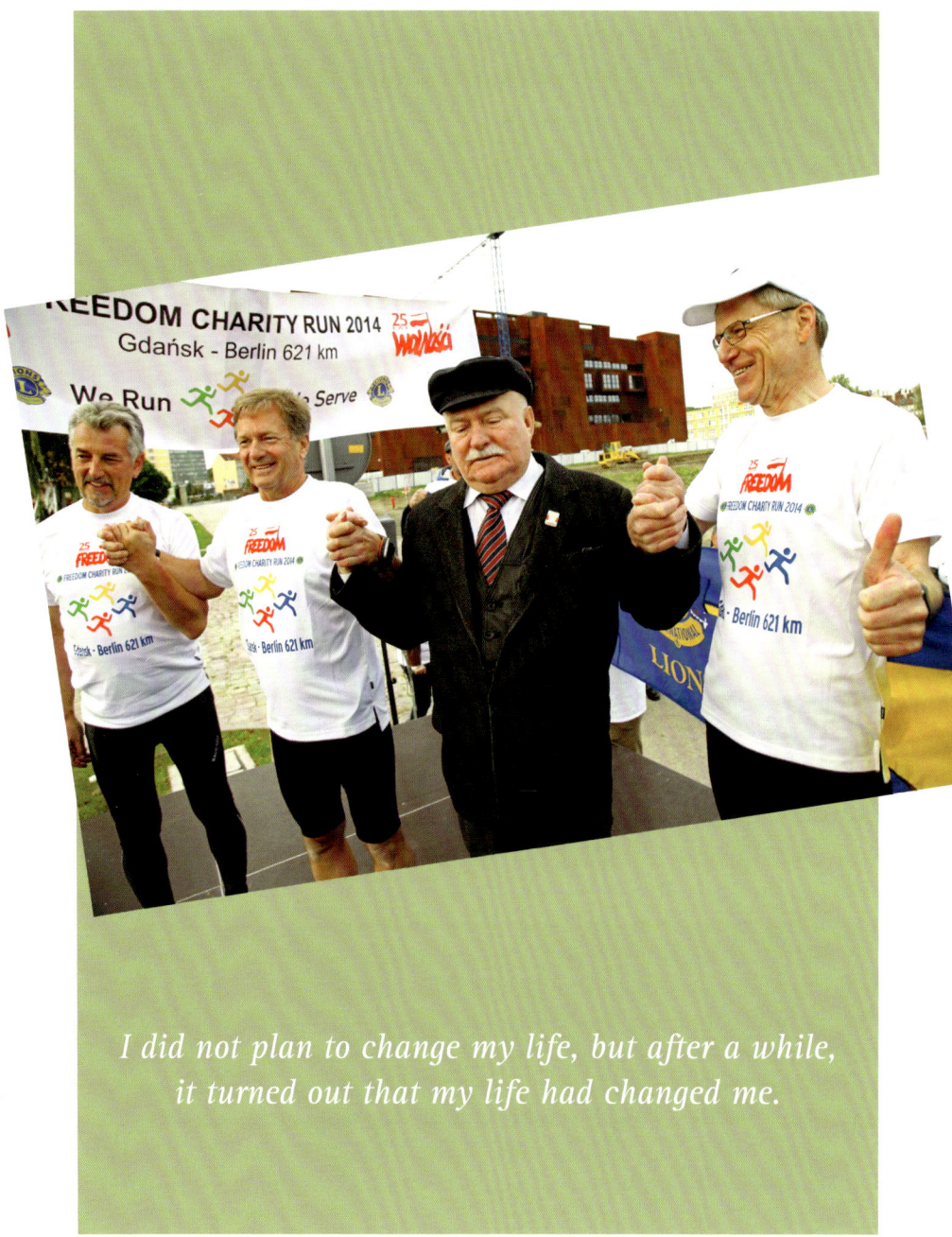

*I did not plan to change my life, but after a while,
it turned out that my life had changed me.*

Freedom Run

Mariusz Szeib

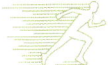 "If you want to run, run one kilometer. If you want to change your life, do a marathon."

—Emil Zátopek (three gold medals in 5k, 10k, and marathon,
Olympic Games in Helsinki, 1952)

When I leaned on a barrier near the Brandenburg Gate in Berlin on September 26, 2004, I was crying like a baby. I was struck by endorphins, the hormone of happiness, which filled up my body like glaciers in the Antarctic. I did not feel the pain of my muscles, I did not feel the beaten toenails, I did not feel the hot blisters on my heels or on the skin under my armpits. I was only ashamed of the loudness of my tears falling on the Berlin sidewalk.

Had I really wanted to change my life? On the contrary! My dear wife and I are happy parents of three daughters and grandparents of Amelia. The company I started with my two friends in 1989 due to the economic freedom after the fall of the communist regime in Poland had been flourishing for fifteen years. The number of our shops in Poland was growing fast, and we started to expand our operations in the neighboring countries.

Ten days prior to my fiftieth birthday, on April 4, 2004, our first grandson Ernest was born. That had influenced my decision. "Grandad, show your grandson nothing is impossible." On my fiftieth birthday, I decided to check my possibilities in a new sphere. I did not plan to change my life, but after a while, it turned out that my life had changed me.

At the time, I had been a member of the world's biggest humanitarian organization, the Lions Clubs International. My friends from the Berlin Club invited me to my first marathon. We were wearing T-shirts with the slogan "Poland-Germany: We are neighbors, let's become friends" in both Polish and German. It was an important declaration in my life. My grandfather and his oldest son, my uncle, were both exterminated in Auschwitz. My father's other brother was killed as a soldier protecting his homeland from the Nazis in September 1939. Seventy-five years later, in 2004, when Poland joined the European Union during my first marathon, I felt an urge to express the Polish-German will to keep peace and reconciliate.

My first marathon was successful in two ways: I completed the distance, and after 4 hours and 39 minutes when I reached the finish, I was informed that my second grandson Mikolaj had been born. The feeling of happiness is relative and, what a pity, it does not last forever. The result that I was so proud of started to irritate me like an uncomfortable shoe. I decided to replace the 4 in front of my result for a lower digit.

I started to train for my second marathon. Running a year later in Poznan, my hometown, all went well until the thirty-fifth kilometer. I do not know who "put" a huge wall there for me, but it got was worse and worse. With tears in my eyes, aware of my defeat, after 4:4:23, I crossed the finish line. Complete failure.

> ### With tears in my eyes, aware of my defeat, after 4:4:23, I crossed the finish line.

What seemed to be a failure turned out to be my success, though. I needed the next six years and eleven marathons to understand it. Only in my thirteenth marathon in 2011 did I replace 4 with 3: my result was 3:55:02. There is nothing like success or failure; it's a subjective feeling that the world will not even notice.

Admiring others, we sometimes feel uncomfortable. Some feel jealousy, but it's a motivation to go further. In a magazine, I saw the 2007 World Press Photo, which was full of fascinating photos. I paid special attention to a group of runners in the desert. "Great people," I thought and started to envy them. I googled the Sahara Marathon on my return home to Poland. In February 2008, I landed in Tindouf, Algeria, not far from the refugee camps in West Sahara occupied by Morocco.

The route was between three such refugee camps—El Ayoun, Auserd, and Smara— and it was not easy. When we started at 9 a.m. the temperature was only 42°F (6°C). During the day it increased by 86°F (30°C). Sometimes strong winds attacked us with tons of sand. Where was the track? The pin-pockets with red ribbons placed every few hundred meters were invisible in yellow dust. A year before, three runners lost their way in similar conditions. They missed one pin-pocket and ran into the dessert. Only one survived, the weakest; he had been lucky and too tired to run too far away. The rescue team found him first; there was no hope for the others.

We stayed for a week in the desert in a sand home with the native inhabitants of the Sahara. We made true friends. While talking, I observed their sight problems. Burning sun and sand storms had ruined their eyes. Two years later, inspired by my

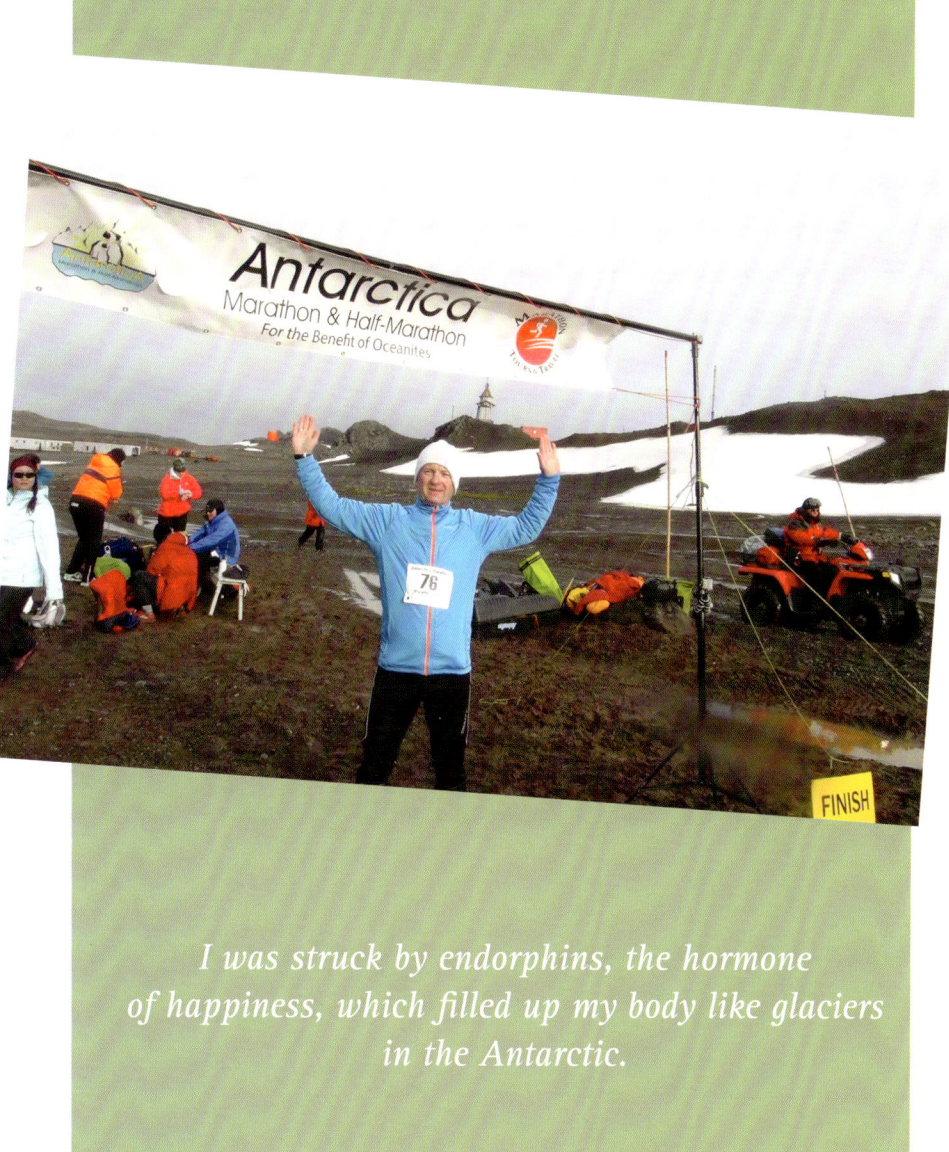

*I was struck by endorphins, the hormone
of happiness, which filled up my body like glaciers
in the Antarctic.*

participation in the Marathon des Sables, a Polish doctors' expedition went there to realize the project Vision for Saharawi. They performed hundreds of eye surgeries supervised by Rafal Nowak, MD, from Poznan. *National Geographic* magazine awarded it the best Polish humanitarian action of 2010.

A double success: doing a marathon on another continent and completing a humanitarian action there. My luck did not last long, though. On September 15, 2008 a hundred-year-old Lehman Brothers bank went bankrupt and caused a series of bankruptcies in Poland, as well. Our company, with its twenty years of success, was also affected. Both my marathon and charity plans were immediately put aside. I had to resign from my dreams to do a marathon in the Antarctic, which was due to take place in March 2009. I had booked and paid my fee a few years before, but now, in the most difficult moment, I could not leave my company even for a second.

It was not until November 1, 2009, when the situation in our company was under control, that I had my first weekend off. After three consecutive unsuccessful lotteries, I received my ideal ticket for the New York City Marathon. The atmosphere was fantastic, and I took another attempt to run it in less than four hours. It was unsuccessful again; I was seven minutes and thirty-three seconds too slow, but I completed a marathon on the third continent and in the fabulous and fascinating New York.

Fighting for the company was extremely stressful. The best way to fight tons of cortisol in my body at work was to run 10k every evening in the nearby forest. Breathless and sweating, I returned home full of energy, and the world looked brighter, spiced with serotonin and dopamine. My determination practiced in marathon runs has proven to be priceless therapy.

I have been brought up in the Catholic faith. Now I decided to thank God for the strength he gave me in those dramatic moments. In summer 2010, I ran from my hometown, Poznan, to Czestochowa, the cult place for many Polish Catholics. I made the distance of 275km in 5 days. I was running along the fields, through towns and villages, sometimes taking side roads, sometimes along the main roads. Although I was running, my life seemed to slow down. I had enough time to think it over; I was distancing myself from its noise and haste, everyday uproar, and race. I felt huge relief, even catharsis, on one side and a flow of enormous energy on the other. Was it the energy that let me run the next marathon the following year in a time of less than four hours? Or maybe did I need a few hundred kilometers of training?

I recalled memories from previous runs. On the last day of my stay in the Sahara, I had given the hosts' daughter, then ten years old, my crank flashlight. "Look," I started, "all the battery torches have light, you have nothing. You will only have light when you turn the crank yourself. When the batteries go flat, there will be less and less light in the other torches. Eventually, they will stop working. "*You will always have light if you to turn the crank,*" I finished. Our life is the same. The run to Czestochowa, although exhausting, charged my torch for many years and was the base for many charity activities in the future.

The solitary run to Czestochowa inspired me to combine doing marathons with helping others. I offered my Lions Club friend, Daniel, a common charity run from Szczecin to Hamburg for the Annual World Convention of Lions Clubs International. Soon, we were supported by a German colleague Ludwig Schlereth. In 2013, Germany was struck by floods. All the funds we collected were spent on renovating four orphanages in Halle.

Breathless and sweating, I returned home full of energy, and the world looked brighter, spiced with serotonin and dopamine.

Since then, we have had our run, now called Freedom Charity Run. For six years, including 2018, we have run over four thousand kilometers in eight countries on three continents. We run under the auspices of many presidents of states we were running through.

In 2014, on the twenty-fifth anniversary of the fall of the communist rule in Europe, our run from the famous Gdansk Shipyard was started by the legendary "Solidarity" leader and Nobel Prize winner Lech Walesa. In 2015, we ran seven hundred kilometers from Warsaw through Kaunas (Lithuania) to Riga (Latvia). In 2016, we ran from Hiroshima to Fukuoka, and a year later, ran over one thousand kilometers from Tuscumbia, Alabama, through Nashville, Bowling Green, Kentucky, and Indianapolis to Chicago. In 2018, on the hundredth anniversary of the end of the First World War, we ran the distance of 1,049 km from Poznan through Prague to Strasburg. We completed the run inside the European Parliament, where we were greeted by the representatives of all the factions with the former Polish Prime Minister Mr. Jerzy Buzek.

Demonstrating freedom among nations and cooperation above all borders is a part of the Freedom Charity Run name. The other part of its name, charity, means helping children in need in Germany, Ukraine, Latvia, and those fleeing from bombs in Syria to Lebanon. We have raised $100,000. We are about to use some funds to start the construction of a kid's dormitory in the small town of Lokhim, Nepal, in the Himalayas, situated on the way to Mount Everest. It is one of the places visited by Dr. Nowak and his associates, who help the local inhabitants save their sight.

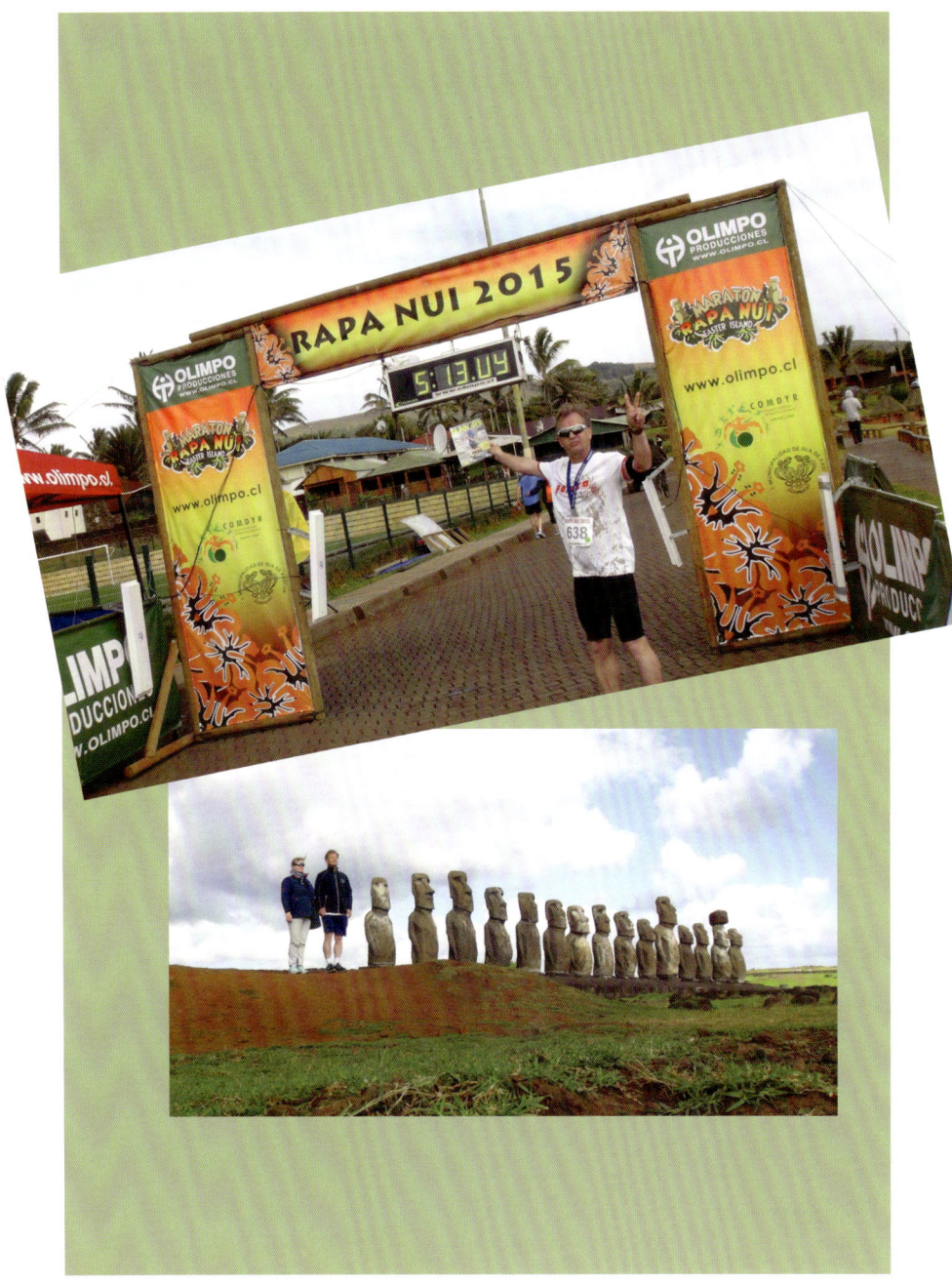

I managed to do my Antarctic Marathon five years later than planned. It was exactly ten years after my first marathon and was the gift I gave myself on my sixtieth birthday. It was there I met many fascinating people like Michael Clinton, the author of this book, and Vincent Ma, among others.

Michael and I liked each other from the start. "I have Polish blood in me," he said when we met at the *Aademik Ioffe*, the Russian polar ship taking us there. We started the run together, we got lost, then ran the last meters together.

While running, I often looked behind. I was not speeding; I only wanted to know where Hein was. Hein was a forty-year-old man from South Africa, strong, tall, athletic and was born blind. Hein finished five minutes after us.

David from Alabama collapsed right after he finished. He had no pulse for two minutes. Thanks to the defibrillator, we got him back. It was only then we realized why the organizers had forced us to insure for $100,000. Rich did not even catch a cold, although he ran the whole marathon wearing only a T-shirt. It was unusual, as the temperature was constant: 23°F (–5°C), but due to a gale (yes, it was a gale, do not confuse it with typical wind), it felt like 5°F (–15°C). The same gale tousled Christine's long and curly hair. They were flying so high that they provoked an albatross to attack her, and she had a dramatic fight with them. Jim broke down 10km before finish. He blamed the hilly landscape, with 1,200m difference in altitude. He had not known, neither had we, that the Antarctic is the hilliest continent with median height above 2,000m, which is a kilometer higher than the overrated Asia with its highest: Tibet and our mundane roof of the world, Mount Everest.

Mike, our doctor, claimed that Jim did not have such hypothermia, as most of us did after the run. He did not, but that day, he had enough of everything. Jim is not a person to break down completely. He did much better the following day, when he ran the marathon distance along the outer board of our ship *Akademik Ioffe*. The organizers accepted the result as a run on the Antarctic and honored him with a Seven Continents Club Medal, as he had already done marathons on the other six continents.

My cabinmate was forty-two years old, Vincent Ma. He had completed 364 marathons which he did in 6 years. In July 2018, in San Francisco, he ran his thousandth marathon. In August, Vincent came to Poland to run in the Solidarity Marathon in Gdansk. Thanks to my charity work, I had met the legend of Solidarity, a former Polish president and Nobel Peace Prize winner, Lech Walesa. I had asked him to meet Vincent, and he agreed immediately. Vincent gave Lech Walesa his 1000th Marathon Medal as his appreciation for his fight for democracy.

I did my last continent in 2016. I ran it five thousand kilometers from the main land in the middle of the Pacific Ocean, on Easter Island as the first Pole, as it turned out later. The route was along the whole island from its capital Hanga Roa to Akkineni Beach. It was where, as the legend written down on wooden plates in rongo-rongo language, in the sixth century, the tribe chief Hotu Matua landed with a hundred companions. When their home island started to sink, they built an ark, like Noah, and set off to find a new land. They called their new home *Te Pito o Te Henua*, the hub of the Universe.

They lived isolated for a thousand years, believing that the whole world had been flooded and only they survived in the Universe. They had a piece of land around them, endless ocean around, and a billion bright twinkling stars above them. Harmony and solidarity were soon replaced with sick ambitions and fights for power. It also turned out that long ears were features of rulers' tribe. Those bearing short ears could only cut Moai statues from lava. These were believed to host the emperor's souls. The size of Moai was growing parallel to the rulers' ambitions. The tallest standing Moai is 11 meters high and weighs 80 tons. Several taller statues were planned. The tallest would be 22.5 meters high and would weigh 150 tons, had it been released from the side of Rano Raraku volcano. It had not, as they ran short of coconut palms needed for the transport.

Through their activities, the inhabitants had ruined what nature had offered them. When they cut all the palms, they not only lost the source of coconut, but the land eroded, and vegetation stopped. With time, their population increased from 100 to 20,000 people, but they all started to kill one another for food, destroying their culture.

A Chinese proverb says, "A trip of 1,000 miles starts with the first step." When I took that first step on September 26, 2004 at 9 a.m. in Berlin, my imagination stretched as far as 26.2 miles. A fantastic athlete, Emil Zátopek, knew exactly what "spell" the marathon casts on its runners. Each of us starts the journey into the unknown, undiscovered land. Each has their own story, fascinating and often kept secret from the world. Marathon makes it real in the second life, which starts after 42,195 steps.

Mariusz Szeib: *An entrepreneur with PhD in economics, he started to run at the age of fifty. He has run twenty-four marathons on all seven continents and is the founder of Freedom Charity Runs, www.freedomcharityrun.org.*

My Years of Magical Running

Joe Brereton

Let me start by stating, I am NOT a runner. Meaning, I do not wake up every day and feel the urge to lace up my Sauconys and hit the bridle trail in Central Park. I never set a goal to run one hundred marathons before thirty-five; it just sort of happened. How? Why? The only thing I can say with certainty is that life happens . . . and we all deal with its challenges differently.

Yes, there are the obvious physical benefits to running, but there are just as many benefits to playing pickup basketball, dancing, or having sex. All of those activities seem to be much more enjoyable than a ninety-minute run along Chicago's lakefront path in the middle of January, when the wind gusts so hard it can lift a two-hundred-pound man (me) off the ground, and the "feels like" temperature doesn't matter because it's so cold you are unable to "feel" any part of your body—which is actually better than feeling the icy needles that were stabbing you in the face when you started your run.

There is no internal force pushing me out on the road on any given day. Running and becoming a "runner," as I said, just sort of . . . happened. You see, to me, running is mental, almost spiritual. When I run, I run alone. When I run, I go "meta" (become introspective). I run when I am happy, and it boosts my mood even higher. I think a lot of people do that. But I also run, and probably more so, when I am stressed, or angry, or sad, or scared or lost or . . . well, you get the idea. This is the story of how running entered my life, how it burrowed itself into my soul. This is how it "happened" to me.

I was eighteen years old when my father died. It was four days before Christmas of my senior year in high school. I remember being in class three days before that when my school's dean walked in to tell me my brother was there to take me to the hospital. My dad's heart had stopped that morning (a Code Blue) and he was being taken into intensive care. While those words were spoken to me by someone else, somehow they took the breath from my lungs. It was as if someone was standing behind me, reaching through my body and squeezing my heart. I'd never experienced this feeling before. I had just seen my dad the night before. He was recovering nicely from a kidney transplant earlier that week. I remember that night, the last time I saw him awake. We were joking in his hospital room, but I was eager to leave so I could go see friends. I mean, I was a senior, and at that age, there is nothing more important than friends . . . and sports. I didn't realize at the time that I would forever regret feeling eager to leave him; that talking to him, telling jokes, wasn't as important as seeing my friends. I simply never thought it'd be the last time I'd speak to him.

> *It was as if someone was standing behind me, reaching through my body and squeezing my heart.*

No individual has the same relationship with a person that others do. In my father, my mother saw her husband, her lover, her partner. My sisters and brothers saw him as their father, but their relationships were all formed in different ways, across different spans of time and different life experiences. To me, my dad was my best friend, my mentor, my idol. He had spent the majority of my life driving me to school in the mornings and coaching my sporting teams at night. By this point, although I was driving myself to school each day, we still evaluated the end of each day together. He would talk to me about school and about girls. There was a time when I wanted to go to a party and my girlfriend wanted to go to a movie. We were arguing about it at my house when my dad overheard us. He told me, quite directly, that I was not allowed to go to the party. Then he handed me twenty dollars and told me I was going to a movie.

We also discussed more serious topics like colleges, and more importantly, which one I was going to attend to play football. Now, before I could make my choice, before WE could make our choice, he was gone. I was on my own for the first time in my life. Sure, I was surrounded by my mom and sisters (my two older brothers were living in Chicago and Hawaii, respectively), but there was no way I was going to open up to them. They spent the early days after he died sitting in the kitchen each night telling stories and laughing and/or crying. I wasn't having any of it. Feelings are weakness, and I was not weak. Even though I was the youngest, I was the one who everyone was supposed to look up to. I had been the captain of every team I had ever played on, starting with youth hockey at age four (my dad coached that, too). I was a straight-A student. I was the tallest, the strongest, and the hardest working kid in the family. I was supposed to do great things. I was supposed to be someone. So I carried on.

I spent the next four months pretending as though nothing had happened. It's actually easier than you might think (initially). I was simply pretending he was on a work trip. My dad always traveled for work, and twice a year, he would take a trip that would require him to be gone for two or more weeks. So, this was just one of those trips, albeit, a slightly extended one. Anytime someone approached me to see how I was doing, I simply replied, "I'm fine, thank you for asking," and I'd carry on about my day. I did this through the end of the school year. My reaction caught adults off guard while most high school kids accepted it because high school is awkward enough—who wants to talk about someone's dead dad? So, I continued . . . and it worked . . . until it didn't.

I ended up choosing the University of Illinois for college and, ultimately, to play football. In truth, football was the driving factor. Illinois was the largest school to show interest in me for football, so naturally when they asked me to attend training camp, I jumped at the offer. This was the first time I was to lace up pads since my dad died. It may not seem like a big deal on the surface, but football was our thing. It's what my dad and I lived for, and he'd never missed a single game. Two months before he died, he was supposed to have a heart surgery. The doctor called his secretary and scheduled the procedure for Friday morning. When my dad saw that appointment on his schedule, he ordered his assistant to call the doctor and politely inform him that "We" play Pekin (rival school) on that day and therefore he needs to reschedule the surgery. That's just one example out of so many why playing football again, and for the first time in my life without him there, was such a big deal to me. And this was also when pretending that he was on a "work trip" stopped working.

I was supposed to do great things. I was supposed to be someone. So I carried on.

The football season was hard for a multitude of reasons, but none more significant than the fact that I had not dealt with the loss of my dad. I felt truly alone, immeasurably lost. I finished out the regular season, even the bowl game where we lost to LSU quite handily, and I ultimately chose to quit the team. That decision furthered my downward spiral. I now had no structure nor anyone holding me accountable. I started partying six to seven nights a week. I stopped attending class almost entirely. And I started drinking . . . a lot.

After my freshman year, I returned home for the summer. My oldest brother was visiting from Chicago and he saw the condition I was in. Not only was I clearly partying, but I had stopped working out altogether. Serendipitously, he had joined a running group in Chicago a few years before and had signed up to run the Chicago Marathon that next fall. He took one look at me and said, "You're running Chicago with me." He was serious. He even paid for it, and he doesn't pay for anything. This is when it began. This is when running, real running, first entered my life. And while my brother's intention was to get me back in physical shape, that would be a mere side effect of how it would come to heal me.

I toed the start line that fall in Chicago having not run more than seven miles at any one time. In fact, I probably only ran that a handful of times before the marathon that year. I was used to just "being an athlete," and to me, running the marathon was just another thing to do—I didn't need to train. Plus, at that time in my life, a three-mile run was considered a "long run."

To be honest, I only really remember one thing from that day: at mile twenty-three, my left leg started to cramp and I was in audible pain. My brother, who had stayed with me from start to finish even though he was well trained and a better runner (at the time), immediately jumped on me. Not with encouragement, at least not in its traditional form. That's not how we operated. He started swearing at me, at a volume that was uncomfortable to the other runners around us. He told me to, "Fucking suck it up and stop being weak," which, at the time, was the ultimate insult. I wasn't weak. At that same moment, we came up on a man running with a prosthetic leg. That was my first *a-ha* moment in running. I was out there feeling sorry for myself, in pain, running a race my brother forced me to run. Hadn't I been through enough in the last eighteen months? Why did this happen to me? Why was my life so hard? Why did everyone else have it better than me? All of these were questions I had internalized since my dad died but never addressed.

And while my brother's intention was to get me back in physical shape, that would be a mere side effect of how it would come to heal me.

Then I see this guy. A man who's lost his leg. Literally missing a piece of himself. Not only was he ahead of me in this race, but he was running with a smile on his face. And there it was. The *a-ha*. The first glimpse into the reality of life, of my life. We all lose something. We all have challenges. We will all have heartache and sorrow in our lives. But we can choose to stand up. We can choose to continue forward. If we're lucky, our bodies will always carry us. It's our minds we have to convince. Running was simply the metaphor for it all.

If you stand still, refuse to move forward, people will pass you by. The world will continue running past you. The race doesn't stop because you had something bad happen to you, or to the person next to you. It will not stop because you are sad, or tired, or because your dad died. There is no timeout. There is NO FUCKING timeout

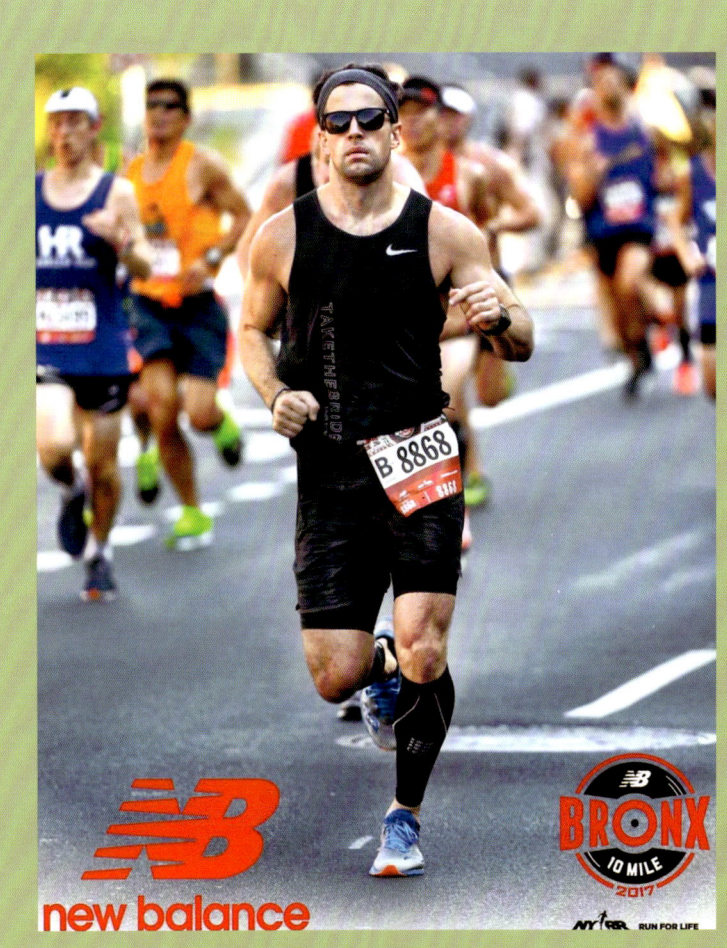

We can choose to continue forward.
If we're lucky, our bodies will always carry us.
It's our minds we have to convince.

in your life! My dad died. And it wasn't fair. It simply wasn't fair. So, I quit football, I quit going to classes. I was quitting at life. But I had a choice. I had the ability, if I was able to convince myself, that it was worth moving forward. To pick myself up and carry on. To face my life, my sadness, my loss. As I said, this is when running, real running, entered my life. It burrowed into my soul. It didn't happen on those three-mile runs, or even the few seven-mile runs before Chicago. It happened when I extended myself beyond my previous limits. At mile twenty-three of my first marathon. Based on sheer exhaustion, I demolished the walls I had built around my heart, the ones that tried to convince me that my dad was on an extended work trip. And when those walls disappeared for those moments, I saw my all fears, my sadness, my weakness. But I also saw my will, my hope, and my strength. I saw what was possible if I was willing to stand up and go for it. And there it was, my *a-ha*. And there I was. And there, in that moment behind the smiling man running with a prosthetic leg, I began again.

But I had a choice. I had the ability, if I was able to convince myself, that it was worth moving forward.

I cannot and will not pretend all was better after that moment. After all, life is not a Disney movie. But that is when I began turning to running when life got hard. It's what caused me to sign up to run the Big Sur International Marathon one month before the race date because I broke up with a long-term girlfriend. It's what caused me to challenge my friends to race when they were struggling with things in their lives. I wanted—I needed to show them that you can deal with anything in your life through running. I've seen friends overcome drug and alcohol addiction through running. I completed an IRONMAN with a close friend six months after he was diagnosed with cancer. He finished in 16:33. Seeing him come down the finisher shoot, and into the spotlights twenty-seven minutes before the seventeen-hour cutoff, I felt tears rolling down my face. This man wasn't sure he'd be alive in three years, but instead of cowering, he had decided to face life head-on because it was one aspect of his life he could control.

So now eighteen years after my dad passed away, I've completed over one hundred marathons and five IRONMANs. I have met some of the most amazing people on my journey. I still run for all those hard times, but I also run for the good times. You don't have to experience trauma to appreciate running. There is nothing better than running with friends while catching up, or finishing a marathon with your mom the day after her sixtieth birthday. But that's another story, for another chapter, for another time. I simply wanted to share how running entered my soul forever and will always be my therapist, my shoulder to cry on, my center in any storm. So maybe I am a "runner." Who knows? But I encourage you, if life isn't being fair or isn't following the path you intended, start moving. Maybe it's running, maybe it's dancing. Just do something positive. Don't stop moving forward, because the race will not stop and the world will continue on with or without you. So, choose to engage . . . choose to stand up. Choose to move. It's worth it. I promise you.

Joe Brereton *has run one hundred-plus marathons, completed five IRONMANs, countless half marathons, 10ks, and 5ks. He finds most peace, training alone on the streets of New York with nothing but his own internal monologues to keep him company.*

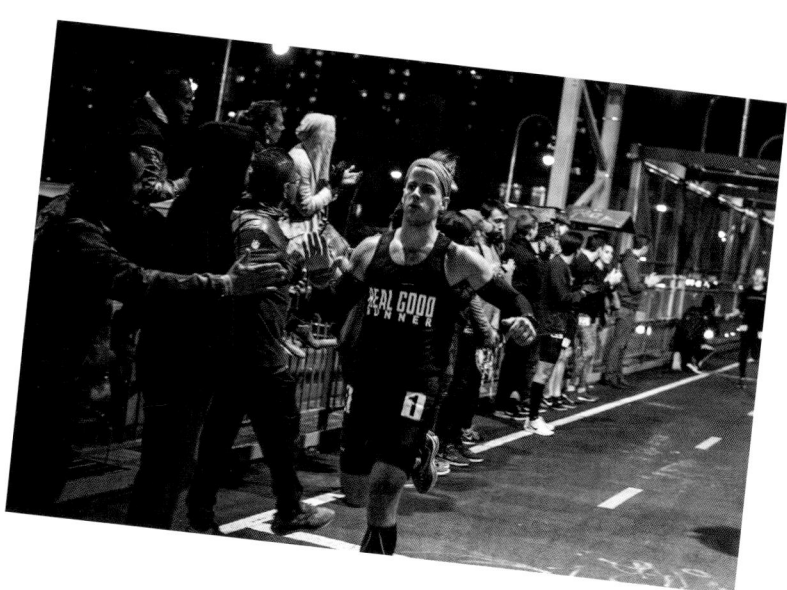

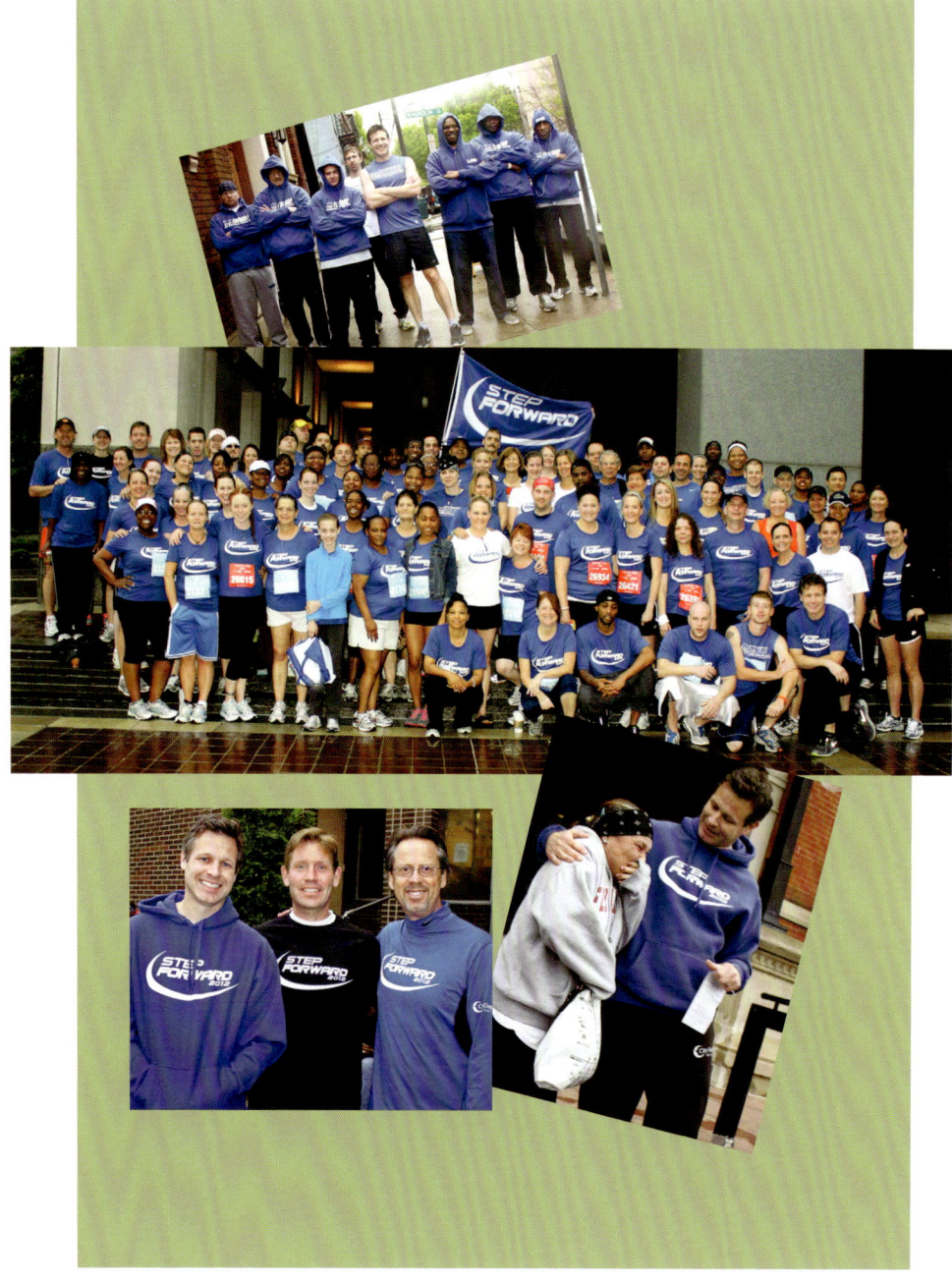

Step Forward in Faith

Chris Heiert

The first one, you just want to see if you can physically do 26.2 miles and still be standing when you cross the finish line. I checked that box at the Mercedes Marathon in Birmingham, Alabama. Then a few days later, I wanted to know if I really trained hard, how fast could I run a marathon? I did my research and put together a thirteen-week training program filled with tempo runs, long runs, track repeats, and forty-plus miles per week. The training paid off, and I ran my second race thirty minutes faster than my first one. While I lay exhausted at the finish of my second marathon, the Flying Pig Marathon in Cincinnati, my buddy picked me off of the ground and told me if I really focused, I could qualify for Boston. Then dedication or stupidity set in, as I pursued running a marathon fast enough to qualify for Boston. I want to share a few lessons I learned from running as I pursued that goal!

Year after year, I trained as hard as the rest of my running group. However, each year after nine straight years (yes, close to a decade), I saw my buddies qualify for Boston, and run Boston, and I kept coming up short of a qualifying time. I was disappointed and discouraged, as I had done all of the hard work they had. I was then encouraged by a friend, Michael, to consider using my passion for running to impact others.

That same week, I saw an article in the Cincinnati Enquirer about a homeless man in Cincinnati that trained to run the 5k at the Flying Pig. I thought that was pretty cool, so I called up the recovery center where the man was getting help, the City Gospel Mission. Over a few meetings with the City Gospel Mission in Cincinnati, we decided we would offer a training program to have men and women in recovery from homelessness, poverty, and drug addiction train and be ready to participate in the Cincinnati Flying Pig 5k, 10k, Half Marathon, or Relay the following year. I really had no idea where this would go, as on paper, it's the last thing I should have decided to do.

I had just had a change in my corporate job, we were expecting our third baby, we were in the midst of renovating our house, and of course training for a marathon is an extra job in itself. But with the encouragement of friends, I felt I needed to take the step forward and figure out how to use running to impact others. God immediately showed up as he brought Dave from the City Gospel Mission into this step of faith. Dave was on staff at the City Gospel Mission and had the interest and heart to partner with me to make this program happen. He and I were going to form a great friendship, as together we would cocreate, lead, and do the work day in and day out to rally the men and women of City Gospel Mission to get ready for the Flying Pig.

I had never trained a group of people before, nor had I ever worked with people dealing with homelessness, poverty, or recovery from drug addiction, and I had limited funds for training gear, race entries, and drinks. God continued to show up and brought a community to make this happen.

The first call I made was to Iris Simpson Bush, who leads the Cincinnati Flying Pig Marathon. Thankfully, the day I called, she just happened to be the one who picked up the phone, and she generously gave me thirty minutes of her time. I shared with Iris what I wanted to do, the impact that I thought the program could have, and how I needed help. The most important thing I got from that phone call was her encouragement as she told me, "Go for it." We would figure things out along the way and see how the Flying Pig Marathon could help.

A marathon is 50 percent getting to the starting line healthy, 25 percent getting to mile 20, and 25 percent the final 6.2.

From there, if you were a friend of mine, you received requests for used running gear, used shoes, water and Gatorade, snacks for post-run, requests to walk or run with the group, and of course, the ask for cash to pay the entry fees. Volunteers showed up to run alongside the men and women and offer them words of encouragement to finish the first training run/walk that was a whopping half a mile in distance. My friend, Lance, was also with me from the start and would be with me over the first four years of the program. He showed up Wednesday and Saturday to help lead the men and women on the training runs/walks that grew from a half a mile up to over six miles throughout the streets of Cincinnati. Most importantly for me, I had my community at home, fully behind making the program a success. My wife, Crissy, and my two girls, Ashytn and Holden, were called on each week to put together goodie bags, sort clothes, and write signs of encouragement. Many people need to be thanked for showing up who answered the call. The City Gospel Mission brought forward their community and staff to help make the program a success for the women and men.

When you are dealing with poverty, addiction recovery, or homelessness, participating in a 5k, 10k, or half marathon is not on the top of your list, so a lot of support and encouragement was needed. Looking back, God orchestrated all of these people to be part of this journey, including the men and women that bravely showed up to say "I'm in" to participate in the Flying Pig.

The Step Forward program was created with the principle to make an impact by showing God's love to men and women through running and walking. In my mind, all of this hard work would impact hundreds of people, and we would have lines of people wanting to be part of this amazing program; however, the first year, we impacted only about twenty-five people. Despite my wanting to impact a large quantity, God was saying and sharing what I want you to do is simple: put love on the men and women who have stepped forward.

Encourage someone else around you in a race; your words may be just what they need.

Getting to know their names, learning a little about their story, being able to talk to them one on one, and seeing them grow in confidence (and distance) each week showed me that going after the "1" is more important than having mass impact. The first week of training when it was cold, there was snow on the ground, and a constant gray sky.

"There is no way I can run 4 blocks," one runner said, but over ten weeks of training, every Wednesday and Saturday the weather and people's spirits changed. By May, you could see confidence had been built in each person; there was teamwork among the participants, and you heard the men and women say "we only have to do four miles today."

The first year, although we were a small team and had a lot to learn, every man and woman that joined and took part in the training program crossed the finish line of their event at the Flying Pig. No matter if the distance was a 5k, 10k, or part of a relay team, and no matter if they walked, ran, or walked/ran combo, each person received their medal.

I was blessed to be able to co-lead City Gospel Mission Step Forward for four years before my job moved me out of Cincinnati. Each year, we grew in number and grew in ways of showing God's love to people through running/walking. Dave has taken the City Gospel Mission Step Forward program in Cincinnati to new heights, as it's approaching ten years of running.

Matthew 18:12-13 New International Version (NIV)
12 "What do you think? If a man owns a hundred sheep, and one of them

wanders away, will he not leave the ninety-nine on the hills and go to look for the one that wandered off? 13 And if he finds it, truly I tell you, he is happier about that one sheep than about the ninety-nine that did not wander off."

In 2010, almost a decade since my first marathon, I returned to the Flying Pig for my twelfth race, still trying to get a Boston Qualifier. It was a hot and wet day that had you drenched within the first few miles. Things were going well up until the twenty-mile marker when my legs started to slow down. I then met my good friends, who were waiting to run with me to the finish line. These guys were encouraging me to pick up the pace and speaking words of faith and encouragement over me. I also had William from the City Gospel Mission Step Forward program join us. He had just completed his first half marathon and waited for me about a mile from the finish to help me finish strong.

As we crossed the finish line, I had William on one side of me and my good friends, Mark and Jay, on the other side, knowing that after a decade of hard work, we delivered a Boston Qualifier (with fourteen seconds to spare).

I went on to experience the joy of Boston the following year and was blown away how the entire community in Boston comes alive for race day. Bravo Boston! Since then, I have dialed back on the marathons, but running is part of my daily life and so are the lessons running has taught me. Running has taught me to step forward in faith. The more things you chose to do that are new and uncomfortable, the more things you choose to do where you are not the expert, the more you need to seek the support of a community through Christ.

Running has taught me to step forward to make an impact. The more focus your gifts and talents are used to bless others and seek God's will, the more you grow your relationship with Christ.

Galatians 6:9 New International Version (NIV)
9 "Let us not become weary in doing good, for at the proper time we will reap a harvest if we do not give up."

Chris Heiert *is always up for a run as long as he has someone willing to join him. He has run several marathons, half marathons, 10ks, and 5ks. He prefers the daily training runs that give him a chance, no matter where he is traveling in the world, to get in some exercise while connecting with his friends.*

Running in Color

Coach Jenny Hadfield

I grew up in a small suburb of Chicago in the 1970s during the Title IX era where the choices for sport for girls were track, softball, and eventually volleyball. When playing ball sports, running was often the punishment given after a missed attempt at a basketball layup or volleyball serve. Running always seemed like the impossible to me. It was my personal Everest and something I never imagined I could achieve.

My first attempt at becoming a runner was less than triumphant, to say the least. For years, I watched my childhood softball coach Rosemary run by my house with a huge smile on her face. She seemed so happy and made it look so easy; even though I hated running, there was something that made me want to give it a try.

Every so often, I'd strap on my shoes and take off down my street, and I would make it to just about the end before I would need to stop, gasp for air, and hang my head with frustration. I always wanted to run, but I just couldn't figure out how.

> *Running always seemed like the impossible*
> *to me. It was my personal Everest and something*
> *I never imagined I could achieve.*

That is, until I did an internship at a corporate fitness center one summer after college. Every fitness center employee ran, and I must admit I found it intimidating, yet exciting. It didn't take them two minutes before they were trying to convince me to run a 5k with them that fall. There was no way I thought I could run three miles. Heck, I couldn't even make it down the block!

It was not much later when my life changed. They not only convinced me to run, but they also trained with me at lunch. We started with walking and progressed gradually to run-walking and then running. Before I knew it, I was running thirty minutes straight, and we were solving the world's problems on our runs. I was hooked.

It took every ounce of courage to show up for that first race. I thought for sure

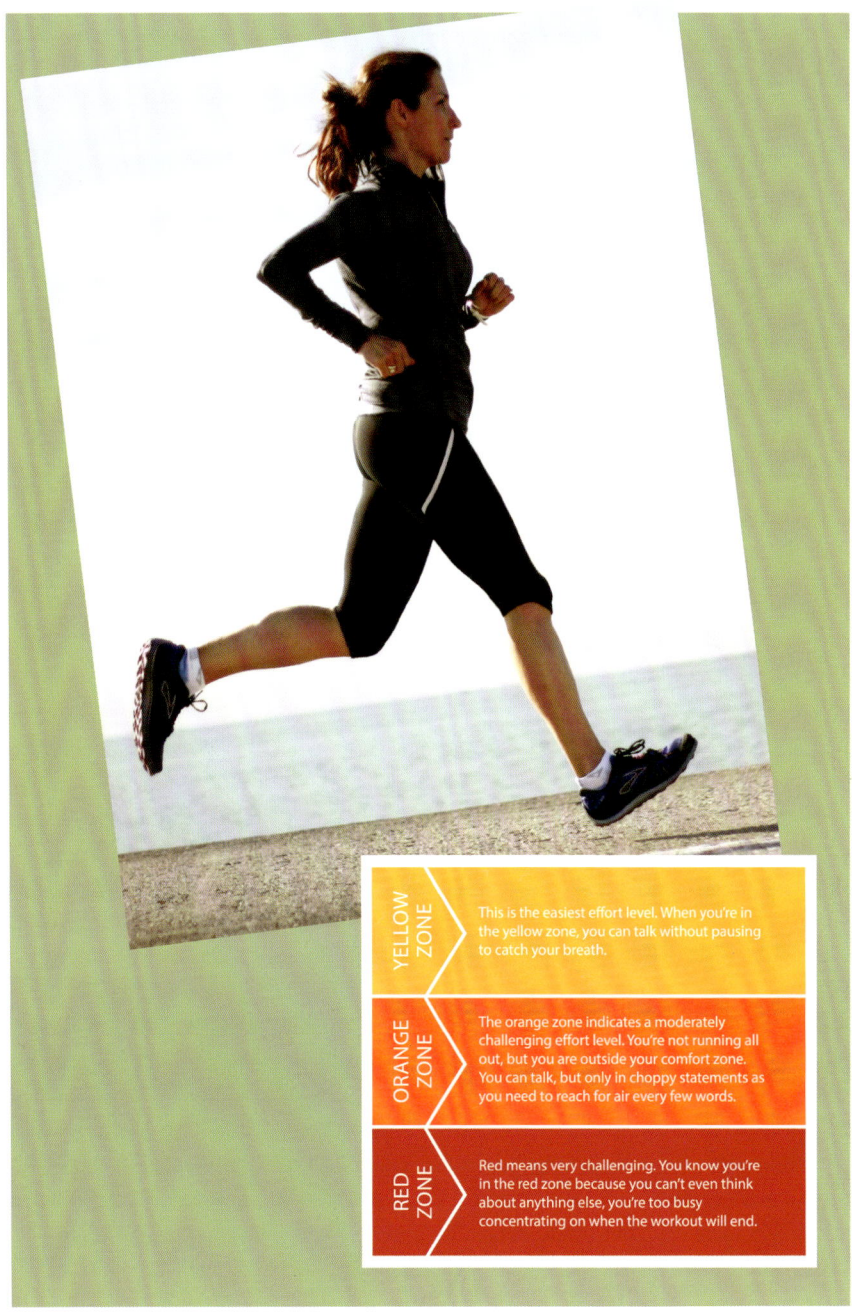

YELLOW ZONE	This is the easiest effort level. When you're in the yellow zone, you can talk without pausing to catch your breath.
ORANGE ZONE	The orange zone indicates a moderately challenging effort level. You're not running all out, but you are outside your comfort zone. You can talk, but only in choppy statements as you need to reach for air every few words.
RED ZONE	Red means very challenging. You know you're in the red zone because you can't even think about anything else, you're too busy concentrating on when the workout will end.

I would be last. Well, I wasn't last, but I was sure close, and was beaten by a seventy-two-year-old man! They even announced it on the PA system. None of that mattered, though, because when I crossed that finish line, my life as a runner began. And it's never been the same since.

Finishing that first race was like summiting my personal Everest. It taught me that I could move beyond my self-perceived limitations and achieve anything I put my mind to. It planted the seed of self-confidence that bloomed into longer races, qualifying for the Boston Marathon, and racing all over the world.

> *It taught me that I could move beyond my self-perceived limitations and achieve anything I put my mind to.*

Along the way, I fell in love with the process of training and racing. So much so that I began coaching others to run and discover their inner runner. In the twenty-seven years that I've been coaching, the one tool that has helped them the most is to learn to run in color.

Run in Color Good pacing skills lead to success. I use a simple three-color zone system that allows runners to learn how to pace from their breathing rate and how they feel.

The Yellow Zone When you're in the yellow zone, you're able to talk in full sentences. Running at this effort allows us to run longer, improves our fat-burning enzymes, and is less stressful on the body.

The Orange Zone This is a step up from yellow and hovers around the threshold at which your body shifts from using more fat for energy to using more glycogen. This zone is the host to tempo workouts and longer repeats to raise the threshold to allow for faster run times at easier efforts.

The Red Zone When you cross over the red line, you are running in the Red Zone or at an effort that is outside your comfort zone. This is the effort where you run intervals, hill repeats, and any high-intensity workout. Training in this zone will improve fitness, speed, and form, and boost your metabolism for hours post-workout.

I have used this simple system to train thousands of runners in person, online, and in groups, all over the world. When you train by effort and follow your body's response, you will always train within the optimal zone on any given day. This aids in efficient recovery, stronger workouts, and faster progression. It takes time to learn to pace by color (feel), but it's an investment that will pay off down the road. It all starts with tuning into your body and letting the data be the outcome rather than your guide.

Perhaps one of my favorite examples of the benefit of running in color is a runner I met at the Cleveland Marathon Expo. Sarah was so excited to share she had run in color in her last half marathon, but she did so by accident. Her GPS device broke on the way to the race, and she was forced to tune into her body during the race instead of following her watch.

She shed a whopping seven minutes off her half marathon time, and what she said next was the most enlightening part of her story. "I couldn't imagine running that fast, especially in the later stages of the race." By removing the focus on the data in her race, she removed the mental judgment of what couldn't be and opened herself up to a moment of personal greatness, running faster than her mind would allow.

So much of who we are depends on what we think, or what others have told us what we should think. Yes, running is an activity that helps us live healthy lives, but it is also an open road for discovery.

My life changed when a supportive group of runners believed that I could. With every step, I erased the fear and doubt and created a path of possibility that has led me to explore my limits, earn incredible views all over the world, and connect with like-minded people. Running changes everything.

Jenny Hadfield *has competed in forty marathons and hundreds of running and adventure races all over the world, including the Boston Marathon, Antarctica Marathon, three Eco-Challenge Expeditions races, and ultra-marathons. She is a published author, columnist for RunnersWorld.com, and hosts a podcast on all-things running and fitness.*

Oh, the Places You'll Go

Paul Gavriani

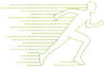 "How are you, mister?" called a small voice near me as I struggled to keep moving in the last few miles of the Nairobi Marathon.

When I looked down, I saw a small Kenyan boy running by my side, smiling.

He seemed proud to be using the English greeting he had probably just been taught at school.

He politely lifted his small hand for me to shake, and then confidently announced, "I can run with you."

I smiled wearily, mentally drained and overheated, as one gets toward the end of a full marathon. Especially when it is less than ninety miles south of the Equator.

". . . Okay," I said, trying to hide my suspicions as to what he might ask for next.

As it turned out, he wanted nothing more than answers to questions bubbling up in his curious mind on a day when so many strangers had turned up to run on the streets where he normally played.

Where was my house? he wanted to know. Did I bring my bike? Did I have sisters and brothers? Did I know there is a dog who follows him to the market near his house? He had many questions.

We discussed these things as we ran—me, a fifty-one-year-old American white guy, and he, an earnest six-year-old Kenyan child intent upon making sense of things.

Besides keeping me interested and entertained during a tough part of the run, this little boy had fortuitously appeared as just one more source of information, one more opportunity to learn, inadvertently contributing to one of the main reasons I had come to this running event far away from my own home.

I am an avid amateur runner and, almost exclusively, a marathon runner, but this marathon, like so many I had set out for around the world in recent years, represented more than just a challenging run in an exotic setting. The race's location itself was just as important—maybe more important—to me than the joy of running in the race, because it had beckoned to me as an impetus for travel, and through that travel, an invitation to learn.

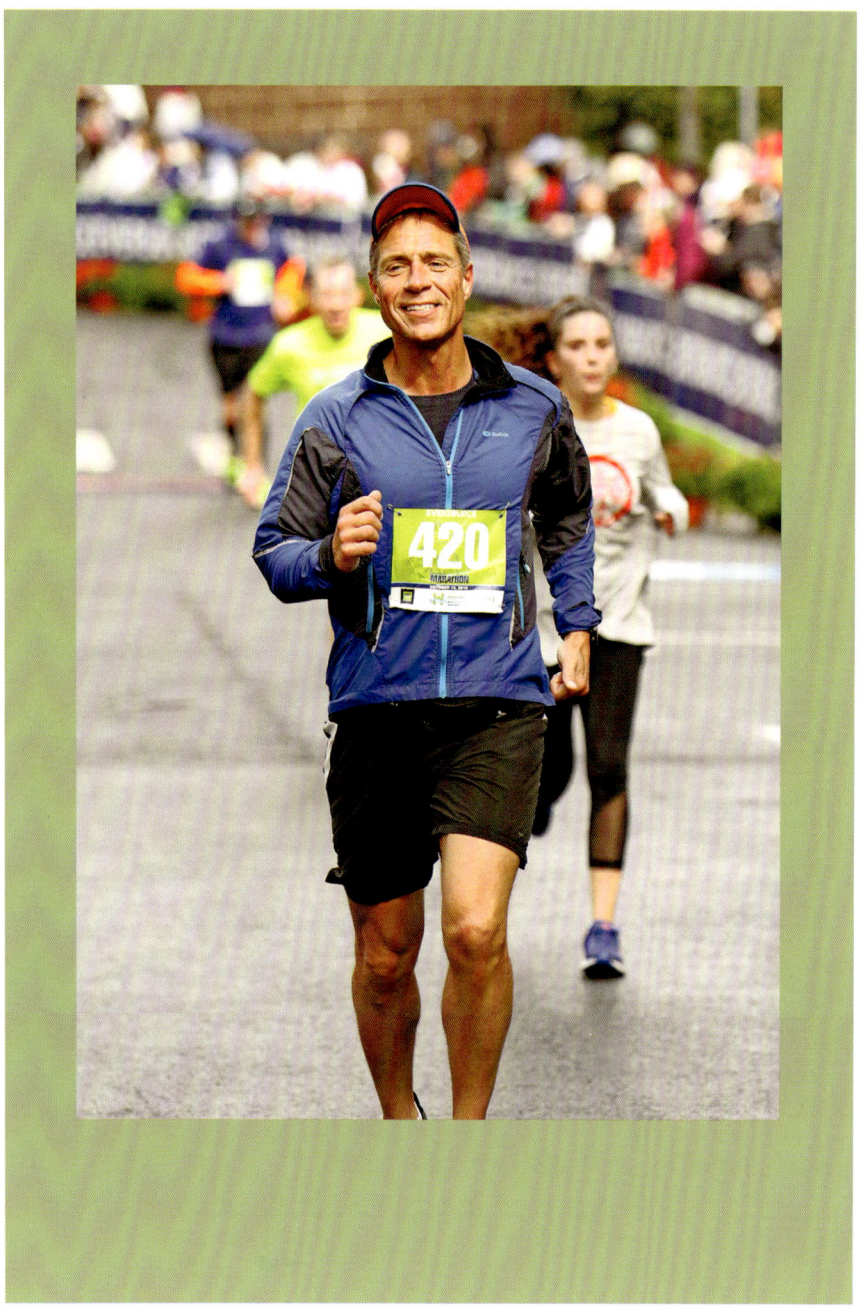

In short, I was running in this city because of the marathon, but in no way had I come to this city only for the marathon.

As I always do, I had spent several days prior to the marathon, furiously learning-by-doing as a tourist in a unique place. I learned about its history and culture; its natural beauty; its food and its traditions.

In Nairobi, this included being escorted on an architectural walking tour, sampling the local food and beer on a nightlife tour, and bouncing around in a safari jeep with close encounters to giraffes, big cats, and rhinos. In those few days, I also felt privileged to meet the residents of one of the world's largest slums (in a program sponsored by a school for impoverished mothers), went on an all-day excursion to the Great Rift Valley, where I rowed in a low-slung boat across Lake Naivasha, walked through the thatch house of a recreated traditional Kenyan village, and was guided through Isak Dinesen's home, the famous author of *Out of Africa*. I even found myself discussing international politics with a Maasai tribal leader, as he calmly led me through an ancient canyon, remote and vulnerable, complete with aggressive baboons screaming overhead.

Along the way, as typically happens on such trips, I'd been a part of so many fascinating conversations that I had begun to lose track of them all; not just those I had had with several one-on-one tour guides, some of whom had as many questions for me as I had for them, but with hotel doormen, Uber drivers, museum guides, waiters, store clerks, fellow bus passengers, and, of course, local and international marathon runners.

In short, I was running in this city because of the marathon, but in no way had I come to this city only for the marathon.

Travel to faraway places has the power to do this. It transports us physically into the heart of a different world where the inhabitants of that place and its culture can be encountered doing their own, different, yet everyday things. Those differences can stimulate our minds and liberate our physical tensions, and in that relaxed state, open our hearts to appreciation, to learning, to joy.

Running long distances can do this, too.

Running, both in its most basic sense as a means of mobility and for the purposes it has served when humans develop it for physical well-being and athletic competitions, goes back many millennia, right to the beginning to human history. It began as a means to survive; runners were the best hunters and were the most likely to survive. By the time civilizations were being established, it was also a training tool for warriors and athletes. Fast forward to the modern world, and what may have been known only anecdotally about running's aerobic benefits throughout these generations is now regularly confirmed by science as also being a boon to positive feelings and mental health. Put simply, running can make you feel good.

In addition, lots of other scientific ink has been spilled to show that when you feel good, your guard tends to lower so that emotionally and intellectually, you're much more open to new things and new ideas.

This openness or willingness to be less judgmental and take in new information can run the gamut of experience, whether it's trying something new to eat, watching an historical movie, or being curious about how people express themselves in a different language.

Those differences can stimulate our minds and liberate our physical tensions, and in that relaxed state, open our hearts to appreciation, to learning, to joy.

So, if it's true that running can make you feel good, that feeling good can encourage you to take in new things, and that travel can often put you in a place where learning about new things is the rule rather than the exception, would it not seem that combining the two—running and traveling—might be a good combination for feeling good? In fact, I would suggest that the combination gives you even more than the sum of its parts.

Consider the maxim that humans are social creatures by nature. We see this sociability in endless examples, along with its accompanying expectations: norms of language, respect of conventions, good manners, grooming and, of course, sharing information by conversing.

Speaking is the way that we most often converse, and most of us have learned to speak from an early age. We eventually grow to see that while talking within our immediate family benefits us, talking with others outside that safe group—literally "talking to strangers"—can offer even more benefits in the sense that we might glean something more interesting from a different perspective.

Socializing with others can also apply to running. While running is undoubtedly a physical activity on the surface—demonstrating competition, promoting cardiovascular health, and elevating mood—I would add that running also has aspects that are inherently social.

Every able-bodied person, no matter what part of the planet they have occupied, has run at some point.

But running can also take place, often most naturally and sometimes inevitably, when people are in a relaxed state and having fun.

We need only look at how children play.

Left to their own devices, before any social structures are applied, little boys and girls run around without a care when they are having fun. If you picture in your mind some idea of childhood, for example, then for most places or times in history in which that image is set, whether it is a cave dweller childhood, farming or sheepherding childhood, Bedouin childhood, Eskimo childhood, aristocratic childhood, or suburban elementary school childhood, you will inevitably encounter children running together because it feels good and is fun.

The fact is that we humans, from the time we are unbridled little folk, into our final days rocking in a chair, genuinely enjoy doing things with other humans. And since running seems to be one of those quintessential human activities universally accessible at any time or place, running is among the few social and athletic activities found in any culture, in any place, at any time.

This applies to running as much as to anything else. We can derive all kinds of benefit and pleasure from it when we run alone, but something even more magical happens when we add other people into the mix and run together.

The benefits from a big communal running event such as a marathon are not even reserved for the runners alone!

But running can also take place, often most naturally and sometimes inevitably, when people are in a relaxed state and having fun.

In a typical big city marathon, a small army of organizers and volunteers, and sometimes thousands of friends and family as fans, and scores of random onlookers, gather in and around a long route, standing outside, rain or shine, cheering on strangers— along with other strangers of all ages—all enjoying the same thing.

A skeptic might marvel at the willingness of these strangers to readily smile and focus their energies so generously on others; to empathize with the efforts of the runners by offering encouragement and assistance, holding up funny signs and shouting out random cheers, dancing to the music in the streets and laughing at crazy costumes. They are there, ultimately, to revel in the feeling of goodwill and social bonding.

This is not the same kind of openness one might feel while traveling to a faraway new place: excited, ready, and open for whatever happens next, feeling a sense of ease, but looking for connections, trusting and expecting good intentions in the care of strangers (be they airline attendants, hotel porters, ticket sellers and tour bus drivers, a museum curator or a life guard), and willing to see how much alike people can be who are in the process of enjoying themselves, too.

Since they are both in their own ways socializing activities, running events and traveling are both conducive to openness, learning, and enjoyment.

If you're a runner and combine the two, however, you get so much more. On top of all the fun in being a tourist and participating in a very social running event, you get the added motivation to train for that special trip months beforehand with the assurance of something standardized and safe in an otherwise foreign environment. You get a definite reason and a schedule to make the trip and the opportunity to experience all the cultural offerings of the destination, and on marathon day, close encounters with the local population who will either be running with you, lining the streets, or watching from windows to welcome and cheer you.

It was something that I knew from experience in doing many of these destination marathon trips, that would serve to make me happy on so many levels, from being a curious and welcomed tourist to running in an event that is a community celebration.

At the time of this writing, I have combined running and travel in nearly one hundred marathons, and I am in the process of systematically making my way through marathons in all fifty US states and in many major cities in nearly seventy-five countries. Each year, I try to squeeze in more trips, so that I now average between fifteen and twenty marathons a year and find myself venturing farther and farther afield from typical bucket-list travel destinations, from Singapore to Reykjavik, Cyprus to Medellín.

Since they are both in their own ways
socializing activities, running events and traveling are
both conducive to openness, learning, and enjoyment.

And because marathons are held everywhere, and because almost without exception, any runner will be welcomed to join in such an event, the menu of options in which to combine running and global travel planning continues to expand each year.

For me, marathons and travel are now virtually inseparable concepts. Time spent in training and in travel preparation is synonymous with self-development and learning.

And yet, you don't have to have been a runner from birth or a seasoned world traveler previously to make this happen for you. I got a rather late start to all of this myself.

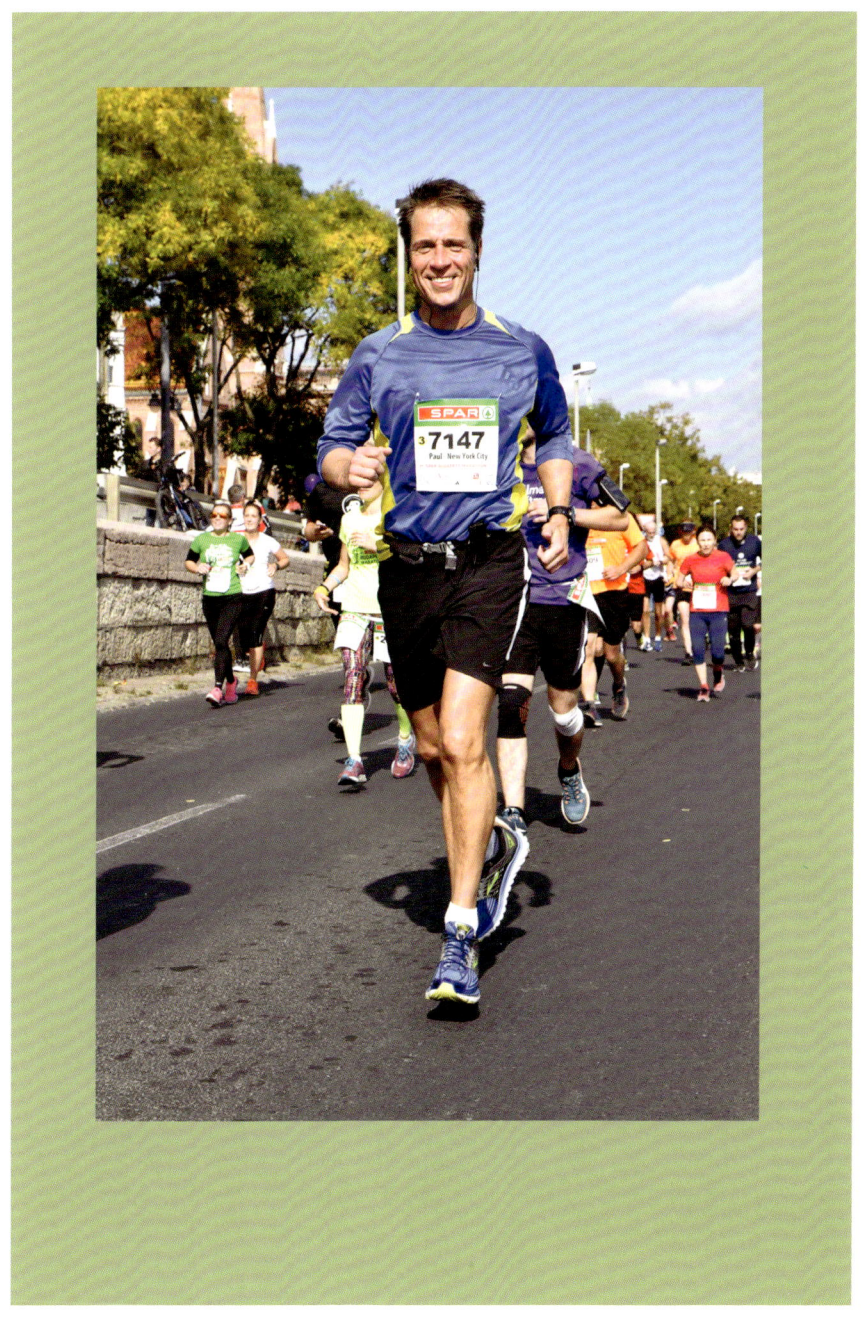

I ran my first marathon in my hometown of New York City in 2009 just after I had entered my forties. Besides looking to get into better shape and hoping for a challenge at the time, I remember that, as the big day finally came and went, those months and months of training that had prepared me to finish the race along with the usual suffering and soreness of a first marathon had not at all prepared me for the humbling awe I experienced simply by being a part of the event.

For weeks afterward, I could not shake off the astonishment I'd felt of running, pack-like, with some forty-three thousand other runners—the excited ones, the worried ones, the friendly ones, the funny ones, the ones who had overcome great obstacles and setbacks, the ones who had raised money for charities, and the ones who had traveled from all over the world to be there that day.

The idea that so many amateur runners had shown up that day regardless of what languages they spoke or from which distant places they hailed, that they would run that day along the exact same course as the world champions who competed further ahead, that they would be made to feel welcomed with no judgments by the spectators, while carrying no burdensome expectations on themselves to win any prizes, that the whole spectacle would be a celebration of something so basic, so peaceful and non-political . . . all of this inspired me to view the marathon as an ideal, a symbol of the happy coexistence that humans can promote for each other when they choose to.

A few weeks went by, and I was still hooked on the enjoyment I had experienced, so I started training for my next marathon.

Time spent in training and in travel preparation is synonymous with self-development and learning.

I loosely set out a plan to run each of the remaining World Major Marathons. Besides New York, these would be in London, Berlin, Chicago, and Boston (Tokyo, which I later would run, was not yet a member of that club at the time). I took a class in Pose Running Method being offered by my health club and afterward found a running coach who continued to teach me that technique, designed to help runners maintain form, increase endurance, and avoid injury.

Since I knew I would eventually need to qualify to run in the Boston Marathon, I next started working on speed with the goal to run a sub-three-hour marathon. I came close, several times, and eventually came as close as 3:10. But by then, I had already started growing disillusioned with the personal best timing thing. Each time I trained for months ahead of a single race, so many uncontrollable conditions would show up and change the outcome as I was trying to define it: torrential downpours, scorching heatwaves, or just illness, stomach sickness, or a lack of good sleep.

I began to realize that the experience of running marathons and enjoying the huge sense of community celebration was so much more important to me than in achieving some new personal time record. I didn't need the marathon to bring out the fastest version of myself, I realized. Instead, I wanted the marathon to bring out the best experience I could have.

Instead, I wanted the marathon to bring out the best experience I could have.

I began to run more races and let go of that pressure to be in the fastest starting corral. But soon I needed a plan. It was already great, I thought, to get some dream destination on the calendar and train toward running a marathon there. I had strategically determined that if I could register for a marathon and get it on the calendar far enough in advance, then psychologically there could be no putting it off until a "someday" that might actually never come.

Meanwhile, I also started to wonder how I could apply some structure to the endeavor, to add some rules to the game. Eventually, in a move that I struggled with before making it public to my friends on Facebook, I came up with a challenge I thought might be interesting to keep me on course. At the age of forty-six, with only a dozen marathons under my belt, I announced on my birthday in 2013 that I would pick up the pace and get in a total of fifty marathons in different destination locations around the world before I turned fifty years old.

That goal was joyfully achieved ahead of schedule, in fact, five months before my fiftieth birthday. But since there were so many marathons I had not tried, so many places I wanted to explore, I immediately wanted to concoct a new goal, perhaps one that would dovetail and continue from where the other ended.

So, I came up with a brand-new plan to run marathons in all fifty U.S. states, in at least fifty different countries, and on all seven continents.

Fast forward and as you might notice on my destination marathon travel review website, the adventure is ongoing. What you might not appreciate at first glance, however, is that along the way I have ended up in places in the world that some people might never consider on their priority lists of travel destinations. But when you want to add Chile, Rwanda, South Korea, or Saudi Arabia, for example, as places to go to run a marathon, you make a point in becoming a marathon-running tourist in Santiago, Kigali, Seoul, and Riyadh, respectively—interesting places that you might have otherwise missed in this lifetime if you were just taking random vacations now and then.

All along, I've felt fortunate and grateful to have stumbled upon the joys of marathons and travel, but I'm happier still knowing that pretty much anyone can do the same thing or something similar in his or her own way.

As for me, it's been an endlessly fascinating journey so far. As I travel to marathon events around the world, I recognize each as a showcase for my fellow runners' personal achievements, all built upon the simplest of human pleasures: movement, exercise, breathing.

It's partly these fundamental things, that make all marathons so reliable yet special. The races themselves may be seasoned with the flavors of the host city's culture, its climate, and its distinctive history, but whether it's in a small town or in a world capital, the basic ingredients for any marathon are always the same: you have people running toward a far-off finish line refusing to quit until they get there, people supporting and caring for them with food and drink along the way, people who are cheering them on, and all of them—every one of them—doing so in fun, in public, and in the moment.

So, I continue my goal to systematically run through the world's great places by virtue of the marathons they host, and as I do, I try to collect as much information about the experience in an attempt to give both runners and non-runners, globetrotters and arm-chair travelers, a taste for them, with the hope that they too will find the joy in running, or in travel, or in any of the millions of pursuits that we humans can go just a little overboard in, pushing the envelope and pressing through to find the happiest versions of ourselves.

When I think back on all of the adventures I have had traveling thus far to faraway places for marathons, I'll always remember the scenery, the food, and excellent professional tour guides I have met in places as disparate as Seoul and Istanbul. But a far greater space in my memories will be reserved for the hundreds of strangers whom I did not really get to know but who showed me some of the simplest human kindnesses: the gruff Russian cab driver who spoke no English and who, without a word, worked hard to find shortcuts to get me past a St. Petersburg traffic jam and out to a middle-of-nowhere race expo before it closed, and then, unasked, escorted me inside and waited protectively to take me back to town when I was ready to leave; the jaded waitress near the start of the Paris Marathon who (perhaps because I begged her in a panic in my garbled traveler's French) softened and agreed to hold my cell phone and change of clothes until after the race because the bag check-in was inaccessible; the food guide who took me on an impromptu, thrilling night ride, clinging for my life on the back of his motor scooter through the choked streets of Mumbai to see his friend, whom he wanted me to meet because she was also a marathon runner; the cousin of a New York coworker with whom I had only met to say hello over coffee the day before, but who then showed up with his whole family to cheer me with a handmade sign at the halfway point of the Athens Marathon. And, of course, those countless "keep going" cheers from strangers on the sidelines in so many different countries, shouting "¡Ánimo!" (Madrid), "Kom Igen" (Stockholm), or "Gambatte Kudasi" (Tokyo).

All of these memories and thousands more demonstrate the simplest of human connections that I witnessed in places around the world simply because I had decided to go there, lured in by and committed to the place because of its annually-scheduled, community marathon event. Those connections, whether dramatic and touching, or just kind and congenial, will stay with me always, so that just like the surprise of a little boy in Nairobi who sought me out on that hot Sunday morning, they keep me expectantly curious and humbly grateful.

As it turns out, the secret in remembering that this is who we are as humans may be simply to recall what it was like when we ourselves were children, happy to run, excited to explore.

Instead of settling for all that we think we know, we must keep exploring and growing as children naturally do, always asking questions, and always trying new things. And even when those new things seem strange or foreign, the choice is always there for us—at any age—to either shy away and refuse to open up to them, or just as we did when we were as unguarded to the world as my young Kenyan friend: run out to greet them with all of the joy we are capable of, knowing how much fun it will be when we discover that the myriad separate journeys we are each pursuing as humans might intersect to teach, to learn, and to join, however briefly, together.

Paul Gavriani *is a successful New York City real estate agent and digital music composer who, in his spare time, is cataloging the world's most interesting marathon locations. Having completed one hundred marathons in the past ten years, Paul's goals include finishing marathons in the fifty US states, nine Canadian provinces, twenty-eight EU capitals, in virtually every country and on seven continents of the world.*

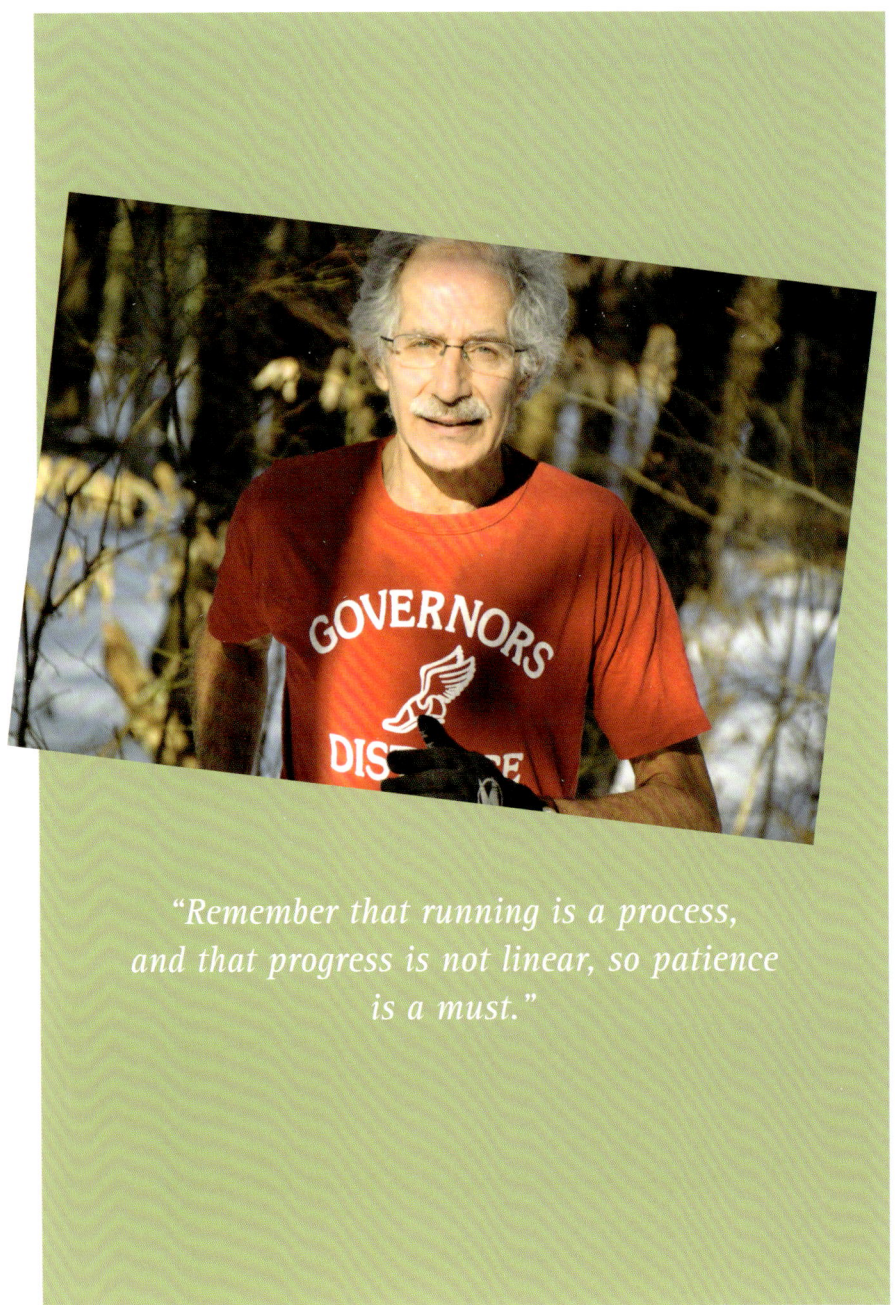

*"Remember that running is a process,
and that progress is not linear, so patience
is a must."*

42 (K) Running Tips

Coach David S. Abusamra

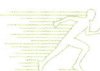

- Run first thing in the morning. Easier to schedule, sunrise, fewer cars, cooler weather in the summer, more animal sightings, but most important, you have the rest of the day to live your life (and to do double sessions, should you want).

- Drink one to two glasses of water upon waking.

- Be existential in your running: define yourself by what you do, not by what you say you're going to do. Think: "I've done 3 of my 8x800," not "I've got 5 of my 8x800s to do."

- Workouts on a track build so much discipline. On hot days, throw ice in a cooler, add cold water, and a hand towel, and enjoy the relief after every repeat. Even though the best rest between repeats is a slow jog, hot, humid days call for this icy relief.

- Accelerations or post-run sprints should be considered part of the workout, not an addition to it.

- Embrace the freedom running provides by not using devices in your ears. Instead, finetune your senses as you run. This is also a personal security issue.

- Run without a timing device at times. Discover your limits. You may very well surprise yourself. Try racing without one, as well. Remember that humans have more endurance than other animals.

- Develop a sense of "play" in your running. Run your favorite route backward. See how many falling leaves you can catch in the woods or how many buildings you can touch in a predetermined amount of time.

- Incorporate backward (and do this uphill) and side-to-side running to utilize muscles you don't normally use while running.

- A workout on a piece of paper or on a screen is not cast in stone. For various reasons, you should evaluate yourself at the time to determine if changing or delaying it makes sense. As well, once you start said workout and realize it's not going well, have the fortitude to save it for another day.

- Most people follow the "hard day-easy day" schedule. Yet, there is merit to going "hard-medium" two days in a row. Or, by following up a race with some timed repeats with a cooldown before and after.

- Add lots of garlic, turmeric, and cinnamon to your food.

- Balance on one leg at a time. More advanced: do so with your eyes closed. Use machines with one leg or arm at a time.

- Fartleks are a great workout to do with others. Take turns calling out the next sprint, such as to the second telephone pole, or eighth house, or third mailbox. Someone chooses the number of pushups or reverse pushups on a park bench, or a backward run up a hill, or karaoke, or . . .

- Run "in the moment."

- There's a cold, driving rain outside and it's time for your workout. That voice inside your head is making up all sorts of excuses. Thwart those voices by dressing appropriately and simply go out the door. Accept the weather (even welcome the stinging rain on your face), and think about the hot shower that awaits. But more importantly, think about the sense of accomplishment you'll get from your "run in the elements."

- Take risks. Do an extra repeat; go an extra fifteen minutes or three miles; do an extra set of burpees. Believe that these mini-challenges may lower your PR by a few seconds and strengthen your mind in addition.

- Run in the woods on snow. Enjoy the utter silence as you notice the animal tracks. No woods? Be the first person in your area to lay down tracks in the fresh snow.

- Oil or Vaseline your legs in cold, wet conditions if you choose not to wear tights.

- Explore new things and evaluate them as they apply to your own body. Calf sleeves, for example. Remember, you are your own person. What others do may not work for you and vice versa.

- As you age, just being able to go for a run will sustain you.

- Continue to do speedwork as you age. This will prove to be more and more valuable to your racing.

- Set goals on three different levels, depending on the quality and quantity of work performed. Identify your weaknesses to eliminate and your strengths to further refine.

- Do progressive runs, as do the Kenyans. Start off almost at a jog, and ramp up your pace every mile.

- When you're in an unfamiliar area and want to run, but not carry your phone, just leave your starting area, such as your hotel, and take each first righthand turn. When you stop, just retrace your steps taking lefts. Then, play with all the possible versions deriving therefrom. You will make fun discoveries to which you can later return to explore.

- Seek out natural resistance training places, such as on sand, snow, trails, and hills. High-knee lifting on snow will leave you gasping for air. Doing your own version of "Chariots of Fire" running is great, but first toughen the soles of your feet over time. It doesn't take long for sand to excise layers of your skin.

- Seek out unnatural resistance training places, such as parking garages, apartment building stairs, and stadium steps.

- It's never a bore to work on your core.

- Your mind is the key to your running. So, train it. Attitude is everything. Remember that running is a process, and that progress is not linear, so patience is a must. Also, remember that running is not your whole life. Try to look at it holistically.

- If you count your miles as you train, try running minutes instead. If you run 7 miles at 7:00 per mile, run for 50 minutes instead. Don't stay in a rut.

- Explore all the aspects of running: cross-country, road, trail, mountain, and track.

- Give back to your sport. Volunteer at a road race, help out at a local school's meet, work with club runners, etc.

- Fast-Wave Workout (from a magazine article years ago): It's a quick, hard workout when you have only 45 minutes and the weather is poor. Ideal for a track or a large field with marked distances. Begin and end with 10-minutes of easy running. Every 400-meter lap can be divided into 100-meter segments. Define "hard" (h) as 85 to 90% of max, and "easy" (e) as 50 to 55%. Thus lap 1 could be 200h 200e; lap 2 100h 100e 100e 100h, lap 3 300h 100e, etc. until the 25 minutes are over.

- Lift weights.

- Log your workouts: date, weather, venue, time of day, how you felt, splits, etc.

- Run where machines can't go.

- Incorporate range-of-motion drills (butt-kicks, high-knee lifts) and strengthening exercises (burpees, one-legged lunges and squats) into your daily routine.

- Search for running quotes (and read books about runners), from which to seek inspiration. Ones like: "Make your own luck," or Shakespeare's "Bid me run and I will strive with things impossible."

- When on roads, always run facing traffic. Choose asphalt over cement; the former actually provides a softer impact.

- Toughen and strengthen yourself with 800- or 1000-meter repeats.

- Barefoot running is natural. Incorporate this first in warmups and cooldowns on a safe area, like the grass inside a track or on a school's playing fields. Then graduate to barefoot repeats, fartleks, and tempo runs, depending on the size of the fields. If you have foot problems, seek a podiatrist's opinion first.

- Transcend the usual reasons for running, such as getting into shape, losing weight, racing your first 5k, escaping electronic devices (and maybe people), etc., and go deeper into your mind to return to your roots as a biped to find that this natural movement can free you and allow you to be fully alive.

A runner since 1964, and at the D1 level in college, a USATF Level II coach of high schoolers for forty years (cross-country, indoor and outdoor) producing championship teams and individuals, **David Abusamra** *also worked at the 1992 World X-C Championships and '96 Olympics. The enduring friendships of the runners who allowed the sport to influence their lives have given him much joy. Aside from a lifetime of tips that he's sharing, he also shared this wisdom upon his reflection of his long love of running:*

"It allows me to return to my Homosapien roots, to enjoy the challenge of pushing myself against myself and against others . . . to seek freedom, to meditate, to work out plans and solutions, to enjoy the comradeship of other runners and teammates, to seek out adventure, the natural world, and surprises, to gain insights about life, training, and racing."

APPENDIX:
SEE
YOURSELF
RUN

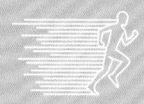

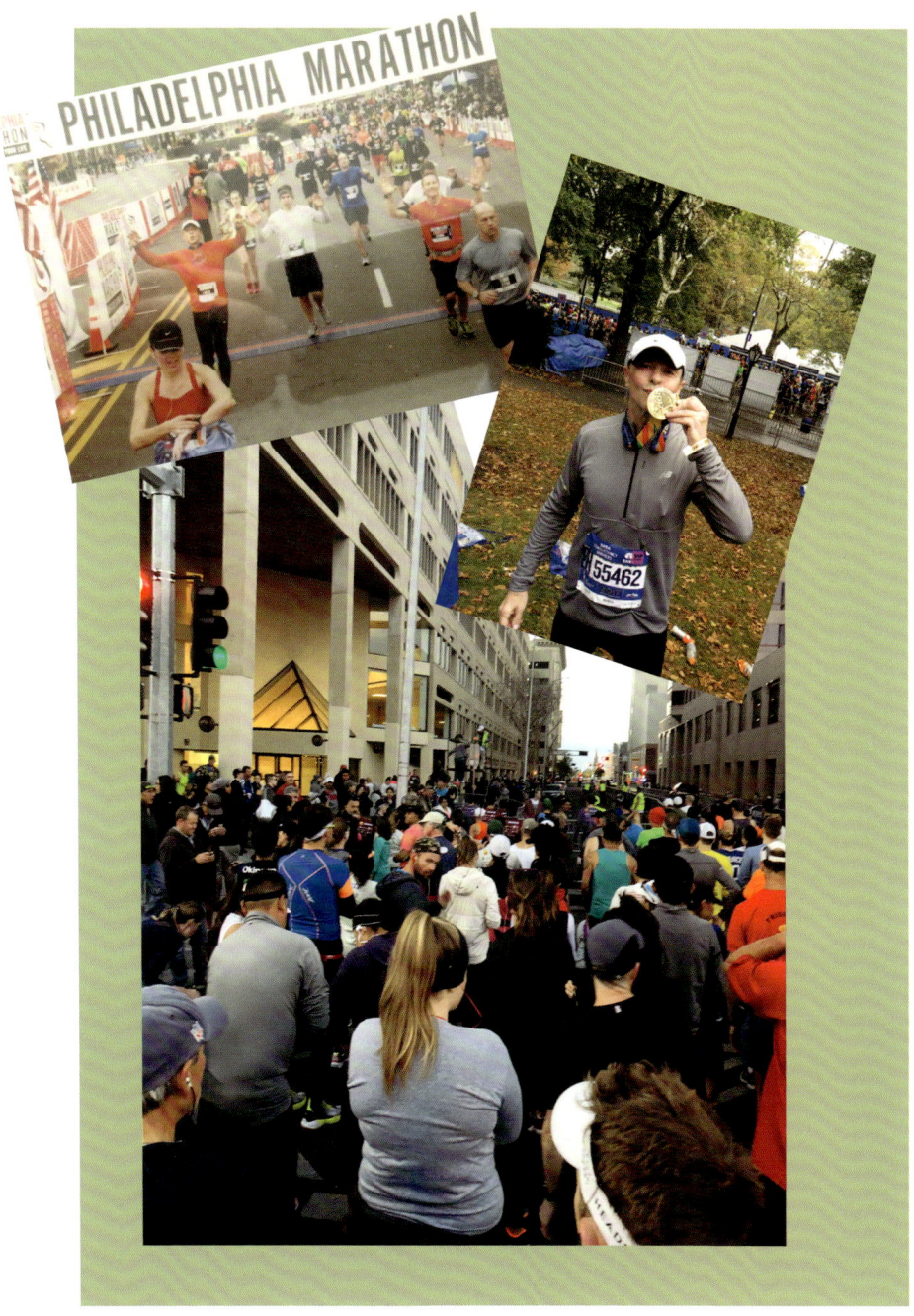

What Is Your Favorite Race?

My favorite race was the Marine Corps Marathon in Washington, DC. The race is incredibly well-organized and staffed. I got the chance to do it on a picture-perfect day, and most importantly, I did that race as a part of the Thomas family team: my sister, my brother, and our parents. We didn't all run together, but we all successfully finished. We trained separately, since we all lived far apart, but came together to have this incredible family experience. Every time one of us crossed the finish line, it was an emotional moment for all of us.

—Linda Thomas Brooks

I think my favorite race may have been the Marine Corps Marathon. It was a beautiful day that started with military planes flying overhead at the start of the race and replete with Americana bands playing along the course, Marines running the flag through the marathon, and the amazing scenery of the National Mall along with the gorgeous trees of the mid-Atlantic. It was also one of the first marathons where I felt confident throughout.

—Keith LaScalea

There is something special about the New York City Marathon. Watching this race as a spectator inspired me to run my first marathon. As a seven-time finisher, who has behind-the-scene knowledge of how it all comes together, I maintain that running the five boroughs of New York alongside more than 50,000 people is unmatched. Runners experience the diversity of the city's neighborhoods and people who all come together for one day to encourage and celebrate their dedication, preparation, and achievement of running 26.2 miles through the streets of New York City!

—Michael Rodgers

Kilimanjaro Marathon in Moshi, Tanzania. Running through the local villages with Mt. Kilimanjaro in the distance was a magical moment. At times, I even stopped to chat with the locals who were cheering us on!

—Peg Pardini

My favorite race was the New York City Half Marathon: the old course that began in Central Park and ran through Times Square and finished down in the financial district. I just loved how for one morning, the city belonged to the runners. All the traffic and the chaos were gone, and it was just a mass of runners throughout the city. It also happened to be my half marathon personal record and where I ran my best and felt my best.

—Gambrelle Snyder

Safaricom Marathon, Lewa Conservancy Kenya. There is nothing more exciting than running in an African game park. The race offers gorgeous scenery and will challenge you physically with its trails, hills, heat, and elevation. It also gives you a chance to enjoy interacting with locals. From the people to the course to the game viewing and the charitable cause, this event is beautiful all around. I value races with a lasting impact, and this event will change you in so many unforgettable ways.

—Kelly McLay

The New York City Half Marathon on February 26, 2017. I ran it with my son on a whim, and it gave me a couple of hours of uninterrupted time to talk with him. We chatted the whole way!

—Mary Berner

The Newburyport (MA) Lions Club Yankee Homecoming 10 Mile Race. Held in late July or early August, you start off heading west, directly into the sun and in almost always sunny, hot, and humid conditions. And it's always hilly. For all of those runners living on the North Shore of Boston, it is a must. It was even more spectacular when it used to finish on the cinder track in the football stadium. It draws competitive runners from as far away as New York City.

—David Abusamra

The 2012 Paris Marathon. Running through the stunning streets of Paris, starting on the Champs-Élysées with dear friends and traversing along the Seine, meandering through the Bois de Boulogne and the excitement of the Rue de Rivoli was breathtaking. Experiencing my favorite city in the world through an entirely new lens is something I will always remember.

—Ilse Abusamra

The 1988 New Jersey Waterfront Marathon where I met the love of my life. I also have fond memories of running the 1994 New York City Marathon with my son, David, and setting my personal record in Boston in 1979 while running the first 16 miles with a college student named Joan Benoit. Wonder whatever became of her!

—George Hirsch

Thanks to the Sahara Marathon I understood that—like the crank torch—we have so much potential for light and power already within ourselves. It was there, in the Sahara, that I managed to organize the humanitarian project, Vision for Saharawi, and gained the inspiration to run marathons on all seven continents. I will never forget it.

—Mariusz Szeib

My favorite race is the Fifth Avenue Mile. It is fast, explosive, and you have to maintain your impulse, energy, and concentration. I remember the great milers of the 1970s and 1980s. I grew up looking up to them as icons of the running world. It is simply magical.

—Vincenzo Pascale, PhD

2010 Boston Marathon because there was not a single spot on the course without a spectator, which provided me the energy and motivation to get to the finish line. The crowds were awesome, and Heartbreak Hill didn't break my heart!

—Joe Suntharaphat

15 Running Quotes and Inspirations

"Winning is great, sure, but if you are really going to do something in life, the secret is learning how to lose. Nobody goes undefeated all the time. If you can pick up after a crushing defeat, and go on to win again, you are going to be a champion someday."

—Wilma Rudolph, Olympic sprinter

"If you can't run, then walk. And if you can't walk, then crawl. Do what you have to do. Just keep moving forward and never, ever give up."

—Dean Karnazes, ultramarathon runner and author of *Ultramarathon Man: Confessions of an All-Night Runner*

"The will to win means nothing without the will to prepare."

—Juma Inkangaa, 1989 winner of the New York Marathon

"If you are losing faith in human nature, go out and watch a marathon."

—Kathrine Switzer, first woman to run the Boston Marathon

"A runner must run with dreams in his heart, not money in his pocket."

—Emil Zatopek, Olympic long-distance runner

"Once you have commitment, you need the discipline and hard work to get you there."

—Haile Gebrselassie, retired Olympic long-distance runner

"If you have a body, you are an athlete."

—Bill Bowerman, co-founder of Nike, Inc.

"While you, and only you, can move your legs from start to finish, no one runs a marathon alone."

—Alexandra Heminsley, author of *Running Like a Girl*

"For running, looking around means embracing the process, including the ups and downs on the way. It means the same thing for life. If the goal is just to connect summits, you'll probably grow to be indifferent about all the time you aren't on top of a mountain."

—Megan and David Roche, running coaches and authors of *The Happy Runner*

"Pain is inevitable. Suffering is optional."

—Haruki Murakami, marathon runner and author of *What I Talk About When I Talk About Running*

"The real purpose of running isn't to win a race, it's to test the limits of the human heart."

—Bill Bowerman, co-founder of Nike, Inc.

"All runners are tough. Everyone has to have a little fire in them, that even in tough times, can't be turned off."

—Shalane Flanagan, Olympic long-distance runner

"You were born to run. Maybe not that fast, maybe not that far, maybe not as efficiently as others. But to get up and move, to fire up that entire energy-producing, oxygen-delivering, bone-strengthening process we call running."

—Florence Griffith Joyner, Olympic sprinter

"Every time I fail, I assume I will be a stronger person for it. I keep on running figuratively and literally, despite a limp that gets more noticeable with each passing season, because for me there has always been a place to go and a terrible urgency to get there."

—Joan Benoit Samuelson, first women's Olympic marathon winner

"Training is like building a sandcastle. Every grain of sand is important, even if you can't see them all."

—Alexi Pappas, Olympic long-distance runner

—*Women's Health*

Michael's Marathons on Seven Continents

North America

Toronto, Canada

Philadelphia, US

New York City, US

South America

Buenos Aires, Argentina

Europe

London, UK

Dublin, Ireland

Berlin, Germany

Africa

Moshi, Tanzania

Australia

Surfer's Paradise

Asia

Lake Hovsgol, Mongolia

Antarctica

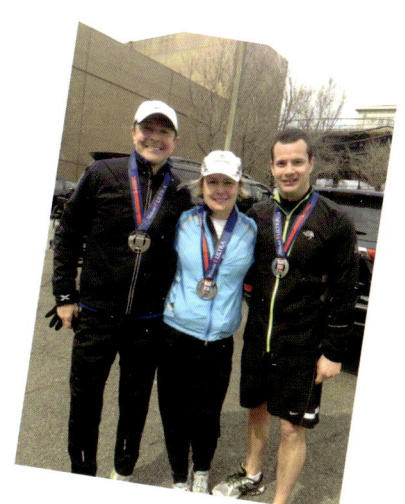

Michael's Wish List of Marathons

Maui, Hawaii

Paris, France

Tokyo, Japan

Everest Marathon

North Pole Marathon

Big Five Marathon

World Marathon Majors for Every Runner Who Wants a Goal

Boston

Berlin

London

Chicago

New York City

Tokyo

. . . or you can run 50 states, all the EU countries, or just a 5k or 10k in your local town.

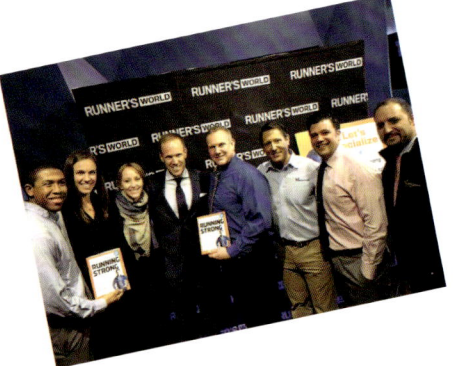

Index

Acknowledgments

The community of runners is a special one that I've always been proud to be a part of. For their contributions to this book, I'd like to thank my collaborators: Ilse Abusamra, David Abusamra, Amir Arasta, Joe Brereton, Jean Chatzky, Lucy Danziger, Paul Gavriani, Chris Heiert, Emily Mingenbach-Henry, Jenny Hadfield, George Hirsch, Keith LaScalea, Kelly McLay, Marc Metrick, Michael Rodgers, Steve Sharp, Joe Suntharaphat, and Mariusz Szeib.

To Michael Capiraso and Dr. Jordan Metzl, friends and runners in common, thank you for the foreword and preface chapters.

For their thoughts and comments about their running lives, thank you Mary Berner, Linda Thomas Brooks, Jose (Nei) DaSilva, Jeff Dengate, Nick Mastropasqua, Yvonne Mendez, Vincenzo Pascale, Liz Plosser, Chris Richter, Gambrelle Snyder, and Chuck Thomas.

To my wonder dog, Hannah, and her posse of friends, Ella, Barley, Buddy, and Buckley, who run in Central Park in search of all that Mother Nature has to offer.

We all have family and friends who support us in our life's endeavors. Thank you to my parents, the Clinton Clan, especially my sister, Peg, who joined me on the quest to run marathons on many continents. To Nic and Emerson, young nephews and future runners!

My non-running friends who sometimes think I'm crazy but have supported me for every mile that I've run, thank you, Andy Carter, Louis Coraggio, Todd Davis, Haideh Hirmand, Jay and Penny Lieberman, Susie Noddle, Chris Shirley, Cap Sparling, Adam Stracher, and Russ Theriot.

A thank-you to Marta Hallett, publisher extraordinaire, who encouraged me to write this book. I'm forever grateful for your support and enthusiasm in the many projects that we have done together. Thanks also to Liz Trovato, a wonderful designer, Rocky Choi, and the team at Glitterati.

Fran Crane deserves a special thank-you for all that she does on her own time to help me get a book out the door. She is my sister from another mister and is family to me.

And finally, to Tom, for the hundreds of thousands of miles that we've run together, I'm eternally grateful that you are always there during the peaks and valleys with the wisdom and pace of perfection.

To run is to open up your mind, body, and soul to the wonders of the world and yourself. There is no better moment than feeling the movement of your feet, as you explore the world, creating your own *Tales from the Trails*.